Houssem Ben Ayed
Mokhles Lajmi
Salam Ben Mbarek

Surgical revascularization and left ventricular dysfunction

Houssem Ben Ayed
Mokhles Lajmi
Salam Ben Mbarek

Surgical revascularization and left ventricular dysfunction

Mortality study

ScienciaScripts

Imprint
Any brand names and product names mentioned in this book are subject to trademark, brand or patent protection and are trademarks or registered trademarks of their respective holders. The use of brand names, product names, common names, trade names, product descriptions etc. even without a particular marking in this work is in no way to be construed to mean that such names may be regarded as unrestricted in respect of trademark and brand protection legislation and could thus be used by anyone.

Cover image: www.ingimage.com

This book is a translation from the original published under ISBN 978-620-6-72839-9.

Publisher:
Sciencia Scripts
is a trademark of
Dodo Books Indian Ocean Ltd. and OmniScriptum S.R.L publishing group

120 High Road, East Finchley, London, N2 9ED, United Kingdom
Str. Armeneasca 28/1, office 1, Chisinau MD-2012, Republic of Moldova, Europe
Managing Directors: Ieva Konstantinova, Victoria Ursu
info@omniscriptum.com

Printed at: see last page
ISBN: 978-620-8-37172-2

Introduction

Coronary heart disease is the leading cause of death worldwide [1]and myocardial revascularization is the most effective treatment for atheromatous lesions of the coronary arteries. It aims to restore blood flow to oxygen-deprived areas of the heart, thereby reducing the risk of complications such as congestive heart failure (CHF) [2].

Chronic heart failure is defined by a set of signs and symptoms indicating structural or functional alteration of the heart. This pathology may result in elevated intracardiac pressures or an inability to maintain sufficient cardiac output to meet the body's metabolic needs during exercise or at rest. [3]. With a median incidence of CI of 3.20 cases per 1000 person-years worldwide, and a prevalence of 1-2% in adults [3, 4]it represents a veritable pandemic, making it a major public health problem.

Systolic CHF with reduced LVEF is a frequent complication of coronary artery disease, characterized by a drop in LVEF below 40%. [5].

In Tunisia, it affects a younger, more active population and has a major impact on patient morbidity and mortality.[5, 6]. CI-related health expenditure is high, due to its direct cost (high number of hospitalizations, pharmacological and interventional treatment costs) and indirect cost (social and professional handicap).[7].

Coronary artery bypass grafting (CABG) is the gold standard treatment for patients with left ventricular (LV) systolic dysfunction with left common trunk (LCT) involvement or high Syntax-score tritruncal involvement, particularly in diabetics[2]. The goals of myocardial revascularization in these patients are to improve ventricular function, prevent congestive heart failure, and improve quality of life and life expectancy [8].

However, the presence of LV dysfunction considerably increases the operative risk and requires a multidisciplinary Heart-Team approach, given the complexity of the decision. [9].

The primary objective of our study was to investigate the early and medium-term mortality of coronary surgery in patients with ischemic heart disease with preoperative LV systolic dysfunction (preoperative LVEF ≤40%).

Methods

1. Study features

The study was retrospective, observational, longitudinal, descriptive and monocentric. It focused on the analysis of epidemiological, clinical and paraclinical data, as well as on the evaluation of early and late postoperative outcomes in all patients who underwent coronary artery bypass surgery in the presence of LV systolic dysfunction. The survey was carried out at the cardiology and cardiothoracic surgery departments of the Hôpital Militaire Principal d'Instruction de Tunis (HMPIT), during the period extending from January 2012 to December 2021.

The study population consists of patients meeting specific inclusion and non-inclusion criteria, which will be detailed in the following sections.

1.1. Inclusion criteria

A retrospective and exhaustive review of the cardiac surgery department's operative report registers was carried out with the aim of identifying all coronary artery bypass graft surgeries performed under extracorporeal circulation (ECG). Subsequently, a careful review of these patients' preoperative medical reports was undertaken to select those meeting one of the following criteria for inclusion in our study:

- ✓ Patients with LVEF ≤ 40%, who have undergone surgical myocardial revascularization under CEC
- ✓ Patients with LVEF ≤40%, initially programmed for beating heart (CB) CABG, but for whom intraoperative conversion to CEC proved necessary.

1.2. Criteria for non-inclusion

To ensure that postoperative changes in CI symptoms or LVEF could be attributed exclusively to CABG, patients meeting the following criteria were not included in the study:

- ✓ LVEF > 40%.
- ✓ Previous cardiac surgery
- ✓ Other concomitant cardiac surgery, such as valvular surgery.
- ✓ Surgical treatment of a mechanical complication of myocardial infarction.

1.3. Exclusion criteria :

- ✓ Patients with LVEF ≤ 40%, who had undergone surgical myocardial revascularization at CB. These individuals were excluded due to the small number of patients meeting these criteria during the inclusion period.
- ✓ Patients whose medical records were lost or incomplete.

2. Aim of the study

To study the immediate and medium-term mortality of coronary surgery in patients with ischemic heart disease with reduced preoperative LVEF (preoperative LVEF≤ 40%).

3. Descriptive study

3.1. Data collection

Patient information was collected from HMPIT sources. For the initial phase, data were extracted from observations related to the various hospitalizations, operative reports, and monitoring sheets from the cardiology, cardiothoracic surgery and cardiovascular intensive care departments. For the follow-up phase, information was obtained from subsequent hospitalization records and outpatient consultation sheets from the referring cardiology departments, or by telephone calls (see Appendix 1).

3.2. Clinical data

Data collected retrospectively for all patients:

- ✓ Cardiovascular Risk Factors
  - Non-modifiable factors
    - Age, gender
    - Familial coronary artery disease: Occurrence of a coronary event before age 55 in men and age 65 in women in the family [10].
  - Modifiable factors
    - Diabetes: Types and classifications according to ADA 2022, poorly balanced if HbA1c > 7% for < 65 years and > 8% for ≥ 65 years [11].
    - AH: According to the 2018 European Society of Cardiology (ESC) definition. [12].

- Smoking: active or weaned.
- Dyslipidemia: Total cholesterol ≥ 200 mg/dl, triglycerides ≥150 mg/dl, LDL-C ≥ 130 mg/dl, HDL-C < 40 mg/dl (men), HDL-C < 50 (women) [13].
- Overweight and obesity according to WHO classification by body mass index (BMI) [14]:
  - Underweight < 18.5 Kg/m^2
  - Normal weight: 18.5 - 24.9 Kg/m .^{2}
  - Overweight: 25.0 - 29.9 Kg/m .^{2}
  - Obesity Moderate: 30.0 - 34.9 Kg/m .^{2}
  - Severe obesity: 35.0 - 39.9 Kg/m^2 .
  - Morbid obesity ≥ 40 Kg/m^2 .

✓ Cardiovascular history

- History of coronary artery disease: medical treatment or coronary angioplasty.
- Chronic obliterative arteriopathy of the lower limbs (ACOMI) according to the Fontaine and Rutherford classification[15].
- Carotid stenosis: diameter of stenosis ≥ 50%, classified according to NASCET as symptomatic if associated with symptoms in the last 6 months [16, 17].

✓ Comorbidities

- Chronic anemia: Hemoglobin < 13 $g\text{-}dL^{-1}$ (men), < 12 $g\text{-}dL^{-1}$ (women) [18].
- Dysthyroidism (Hypothyroidism, Hyperthyroidism).
- Supraventricular rhythm disorder (atrial fibrillation (AF), atrial flutter).
- Peptic ulcer.
- Transient ischemic attack (TIA) or cerebrovascular accident (CVA).
- Chronic obstructive pulmonary disease (COPD).
- Chronic renal failure (CRF) according to the K/DOQI classification [19] (Table 1).

Table 1 Classification of stages of chronic kidney disease

STADE	GFR (ml/min/1.73 m2)	Definition
1	≥ 90	CKD* with normal or increased GFR
2	Between 60 and 89	MRC* with slightly reduced GFR
3A	Between 45 and 59	Moderate CKD
3B	Between 30 and 44	
4	Between 15 and 29	Severe CKD
5	< 15	End-stage CKD

CKD: Chronic kidney disease, **GFR:** Glomerular filtration rate,
CKD: chronic renal failure. * proteinuria, abnormalities on renal imaging, or anatomopathological abnormalities

✓ Reason for hospitalization

- Unstable angina.
- Acute coronary syndrome (ACS) without persistent ST-segment elevation and elevated troponins (NSTEMI).
- Progressive ACS with persistent ST-segment elevation (STEMI) (< 48 hours).
- STEMI seen late (>48 hours).
- Chronic coronary syndrome:
  - Stable angina.
  - Assessment of ischemic cardiomyopathy or LV dysfunction diagnosed on transthoracic echocardiography (TTE).
  - Silent ischemia revealed by myocardial ischemia scintigraphy or stress or stress echocardiography.
- Degree of surgical urgency: emergency or scheduled surgery.
- The presence or absence of a critical preoperative state, defined according to Euroscore II criteria [20-22]by the presence of at least one of the following preoperative parameters:
  - Presence of ventricular tachycardia.
  - Placement of an intraaortic counterpulsation balloon (BCPIA).
  - Cardiorespiratory arrest recovered.
  - Cardiac massage.

- Mechanical ventilation.
- Vasopressors.
- Acute renal failure.

o Patients' functional discomfort was assessed according to the New York Heart Association (NYHA) classification before CABG (the most pessimistic) and during follow-up (the most optimistic) [23] (Appendix 2).

3.3. Data paraclinical

3.3.1. Biology

Relevant information was collected, including: pre- and postoperative blood creatinine values, creatinine clearances calculated according to the Cockcroft and Gault formula [24]pre- and postoperative hemoglobin values, hematocrit, white blood cells, platelets, LDL cholesterol, HDL cholesterol, triglycerides, fasting blood glucose, HbA1c, troponin levels, liver function tests, ABO and Rhesus blood groups.

3.3.2. Electrocardiogram data

An electrocardiogram was performed in all patients to look for :

- ✓ Heart rhythm disorders.
- ✓ Atrioventricular conduction disorders.
- ✓ Disorders of ventricular excitability.
- ✓ Sequelae of myocardial necrosis.
- ✓ Repolarization disorders.

3.3.3. Data from resting transthoracic echocardiography

The above data were collected from echocardiography reports preoperatively, postoperatively and during follow-up.

- ✓ LV systolic function: LVEF assessed by the Simpson biplane method. This LVEF was considered reduced if it was less than 40%. [3].
- ✓ Disorders of LV segmental kinetics: These disorders have been classified as hypokinesia, akinesia or dyskinesia for each myocardial segment. For the latter, the segmentation of the American Society of Echocardiography has been adopted [25].

- ✓ Systolic pulmonary arterial pressures (SPAPs): SPAP values were extracted from pre-existing echocardiography reports and classified into two categories, in accordance with Euroscore II criteria [22]
  - o Between 31 and 55 mmHg: Average rise in PAPS.
  - o > 55 mmHg: Severe elevation of PAPS.
- ✓ Valvular status: presence of associated valvular disease, notably functional mitral insufficiency (MI) of ischemic origin.
- ✓ Evaluation of the left atrial surface.
- ✓ Search for left intraventricular thrombus.
- ✓ Right ventricular systolic function.

3.3.4. Doppler ultrasound data of the supra aortic trunks

Search for associated carotid atheromatous lesions and their hemodynamic severity.

3.3.5. Data coronary angiography

The various coronary lesions were analyzed:

- ✓ Seat of stenosis: This has been defined with reference to the classification of the American College of Cardiology and the American Heart Association (ACC/AHA).[26].
- ✓ Patients were classified as mono-, bi- or tritruncular, depending on whether the main axes (anterior interventricular artery (IVA), circumflex artery (Cx) or right coronary artery (CD)) or their collaterals (diagonal artery (Dg), marginal artery (Mg), posterior interventricular artery (IVP) or left retroventricular artery (RVG)) were involved.
- ✓ Severity of stenosis :
  - o A stenosis was considered significant if it was ≥ 50% at the level of the TCG, or at the level of the ostial IVA, and ≥ 70% at the level of other arteries of diameter ≥2 millimeters (mm).
  - o A chronic coronary occlusion corresponds to a complete interruption of the anterograde blood flow of a coronary artery, and on coronary angiography it corresponds to a TIMI 0 (Thrombolysis In Myocardial Infarction) flow[27]. This obstruction must have been present for at least three months.

- Coronary flow analysis: A classification developed by the TIMI study team distinguished 4 types of flow (14) (Appendix 3).

✓ The SYNTAX Score I anatomical risk score was not calculated due to lack of data.

3.3.6. Myocardial scintigraphy or dobutamine echocardiography

These examinations were performed either to document myocardial ischemia or to verify the viability of a systematized territory of a coronary artery in order to justify its revascularization.

3.4. Calculation of predictive scores for early mortality

3.4.1. Euroscore II

It was developed by the European Association of Cardiothoracic Surgeons to assess surgical risk. Euroscore II is currently the most widely used (Appendix 5). It was updated in 2011. It is more precise for patients with comorbidities. It is a predictive score of in-hospital mortality for cardiac surgery [20].

3.4.2. STS Risk Score

It was developed by "The Society of thoracic surgeons' risk score" to predict surgical morbidity and mortality.[28]. It is based on data from the National Adult Cardiac Surgery Database (Appendix 6).

3.5. Treatment strategy

The therapeutic decision of the medical-surgical team was retrospectively analyzed on the basis of observations and collegial decisions recorded manually in the patient's various medical records. This analysis identified the following parameters.

- ✓ Degree of urgency.
- ✓ Management delay: Time between the date of the CABG and the date of the coronary angiography in days
- ✓ Approach: vertical median sternotomy
- ✓ Type of procedure: under CEC after general heparinization, followed by cannulation of the ascending aorta and right atrium.
- ✓ Bypass surgery

- o The type of grafts used: arterial or venous
- o Revascularized arteries,
- o Number of bridges, number of distal anastomoses
- o Type of anastomosis of the right internal mammary artery (AMID): pedicled by tunnelling through the sinus of Theile, as a free Y-mounted graft on the left internal mammary artery (AMIG).
- o Types of sequential PAC.

- ✓ Duration of bypass surgery, aortic clamping, circulatory assistance
- ✓ CEC discharge: easy or having required positive inotropic drugs, "Levosimendan", and/or BCPIA in case of low cardiac output syndrome (SBDC).
- ✓ Timing of BCPIA insertion: pre-, intra- or postoperative
- ✓ Type of revascularization: complete or incomplete. Revascularization was considered complete when all bypasses were performed on arteries with a stenosis deemed significant on the basis of preoperative angiographic data.
- ✓ Duration of mechanical ventilation in hours.
- ✓ Length of stay in intensive care

3.6. Early post-operative results

3.6.1. Early postoperative mortality:

Early mortality is defined as any death occurring within 30 days of surgery or during hospitalization, whether in the cardiovascular resuscitation department or after transfer to the cardiology department.

3.6.2. Complications early post-operative

Early postoperative complications (between D0 and D30) were noted:

- ✓ STROKE/TIA.
- ✓ Myocardial infarction (MI) type 5: iatrogenic MI after coronary artery bypass grafting (CABG) defined by a troponin elevation of more than 10 times the normal value, or more than 20% for patients with an elevated but stable troponin value associated with at least one of the following signs [29] :
    - ▪ Symptoms of acute myocardial ischemia.
    - ▪ Dynamic ECG changes or appearance of pathological Q waves.

- Appearance of abnormal segmental kinetics or myocardial viability on imaging.

- ✓ Post-operative low cardiac output syndrome (LCAS) is defined as dysfunction of the heart's pumping function, resulting in reduced systemic perfusion and potentially leading to tissue hypoxia and organ failure. Generally transient and responsive to conventional medical treatment, it may become refractory and require mechanical circulatory support. In the literature, SBDC is commonly defined by a decrease in cardiac output (below 2.2 L/min/m²) with signs of hypoperfusion (excluding hypovolemia), the need for two inotropic drugs postoperatively, or the need for mechanical circulatory support to exit bypass or postoperatively[30].
- ✓ Infectious complications: acute mediastinitis and its delay, infectious pneumonitis, urinary tract infection, septicemia, medical device infection.
- ✓ Hemorrhagic complications with or without revisional hemostasis surgery.
- ✓ Respiratory complications.
- ✓ Postoperative acute renal failure.

We determined early major cardiovascular events (MACCE), which were defined by the occurrence within 30 days of the revascularization procedure of:

- ✓ Early death.
- ✓ Type 5 myocardial infarction.
- ✓ Post-operative stroke.
- ✓ SBDC.

3.7. Late follow-up

Late follow-up was carried out at the cardiology outpatient clinic after consulting the records or by telephone calls.

We recorded various out-of-hospital complications, functional symptomatology, and left ventricular function by transthoracic echocardiography.

Late death was defined as death within 30 days of surgery.

Late MACCE was defined as the occurrence of late death, stroke or coronary syndromes after 30 days of surgery.

If angiographic monitoring was required following postoperative MACCE, information concerning coronary angiography and the treatment strategy adopted was meticulously recorded and reported.

4. Analytical study:

The aim of this phase of the study was to investigate factors predictive of early and late mortality, as well as those associated with early and late major cardiovascular complications after surgery. Predictors of postoperative complications associated with death were also investigated.

A further analysis sought to identify factors predictive of deterioration in LVEF recorded early postoperatively and during follow-up.

Finally, an analysis of overall survival and the period free of major cardiovascular complications was carried out.

5. Statistical analysis

It was conducted using IBM software® SPSS-statistic® version 28 for macOS with license and EasyMedStat online automated statistics software (version 3.24; www.easymedstat.com) for a fee.

5.1. Descriptive study

In the first stage of the analysis, the study population was described in terms of all the variables collected. For qualitative variables, simple and relative frequencies were calculated, while for quantitative variables, means, medians and standard deviations were determined. Results following a normal distribution were expressed as mean ± standard deviation, and those not following this distribution were represented by the median and interquartile range. Conformity of the sample to the normal distribution was confirmed using the Shapiro-Wilk and K-S tests, and the following statistical methods were applied.

5.1.1. Comparison of categorical variables

The comparison of the two percentages on independent series was carried out using Pearson'sχ 2 test. When the size of one of the groups was less than 5, the results of Fisher's two-tailed exact test were used instead. A significance level of 5.0% (two-tailed) was set.

5.1.2. Comparison of quantitative variables

Comparisons of two means on independent series were carried out using Student's t-test. In the case of small numbers or non-normality of distribution, the non-parametric Mann-Whitney test was chosen.

Comparisons of several means on independent series were carried out using the one-factor ANOVA test or, in the event of non-normality or small numbers, the non-parametric Kruskal-Wallis test.

The correlation between two quantitative variables was determined by Pearson's correlation coefficient, if they validated normality, or by Spearman's non-parametric rank correlation coefficient test, if they did not. Results were presented in tabular or graphical form, making them easier to interpret and understand.

5.2. Analytical study

5.2.1. Searching for risk factors

5.2.1.1. Study univariate

Risk factors were identified by calculating the Odds Ratio (OR) and its confidence interval. The OR indicates how many times the risk of an event is multiplied when there is exposure to a factor compared with non-exposure.

To calculate the ORs of the quantitative variables, these were transformed into two-modality qualitative variables. The distribution threshold of the quantitative variable was determined using ROC curves (Receiver Operating Curves). After checking that the area under the curve was significantly greater than 0.50, the threshold was chosen based on the value of the variable offering the best sensitivity and specificity, in accordance with Youden's point.

OR results will be transcribed using the following format OR= *Value* (IC95% minimum value; IC95% maximum value), *p=value*.

5.2.1.2. Study multivariate

Multivariate analysis was performed only when the number of individuals per group exceeded 30, using stepwise top-down logistic regression. Dependent variables studied included overall mortality, MACCE onset, postoperative LVEF impairment and renal

function impairment. The explanatory variables selected included prognostic factors identified in the pre-existing literature, as well as those retained by our univariate analysis, with significance set at $p < 0.25$. Model fit was validated using the Hosmer Lemeshow test, with a significance level set at 0.05. The predictive power of the model was assessed by Nagelkerke's R-squared and the concordance index, or "C statistic". The alpha risk was set at 5%. Patients with missing data were excluded from the analysis.
For the quantitative variables analyzed, multivariate linear regression was performed to assess the relationship between this variable and the explanatory variables. Data were checked for multicollinearity using the Belsley-Kuh-Welsch technique. Residuals were tested for heteroscedasticity and normality using the Breusch-Pagan and Shapiro-Wilk tests respectively. A p-value < 0.05 was considered statistically significant. Missing data for some explanatory variables were imputed by the mean for numerical variables and the most frequent modality for discrete variables. Patients with more than five percent missing data were excluded from the analysis. Newey West correction for heteroscedasticity was applied. Multivariate analysis was performed with EasyMedStat (version 3.27; www.easymedstat.com).

5.2.1.3. Survival analysis

Survival data were studied by establishing survival curves using the "Kaplan Meier" method. The search for prognostic factors for survival was carried out in univariate analysis (factor by factor) by comparing the survival curves using the "Log Rank" test. We also expressed their Hazard Ratio (HR) and 95% CI. The alpha risk was set at 5.0%. Multivariate Cox regression was performed to assess relationships between explanatory variables. Data were checked for multicollinearity using the Belsley-Kuh-Welsch technique, and proportional hazards were checked against Schoenfeld residuals. The alpha risk was set at 5%. Statistical analysis was performed with EasyMedStat (version 3.27; www.easymedstat.com).

6. Bibliographic research

The bibliographic search was carried out on the "Pubmed", "Google Scholar", "Research Gate", "Wiley Online Library" and "Science Direct" platforms.

Using the predefined keywords from the thesis: cardiac surgery, left ventricular dysfunction, coronary bypass surgery, prognosis . We also associated the different scores and complications and the different types of surgery in the search.

We have then selected the most relevant and recent articles for reference.

Endnote® 21 for macOS was used to manage bibliographic references in a Vancouver style adapted to the recommendations of the Tunis Faculty of Medicine.

7. Conflicts of interest

It should also be noted that there were no ethical considerations or conflicts of interest during the preparation of this work.

Results

1. Patient recruitment

In the decade between January 2012 and December 2021, 819 patients underwent isolated myocardial revascularization surgery. The preoperative medical records of all these patients were reviewed, revealing 77 patients with an LVEF below 40%. Of these, 76 were initially scheduled for CEC surgery, while one patient, initially scheduled for CB surgery, underwent intraoperative conversion to CEC. Four medical records were missing or incomplete, leading to the exclusion of these patients from the study.

The file recruitment process for our study is summarized in Figure 1.

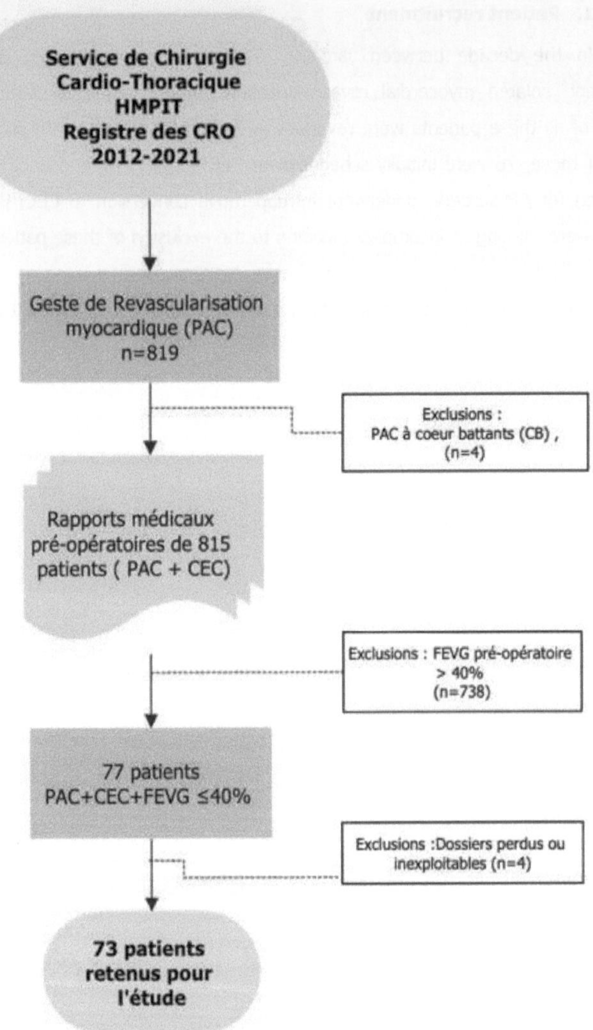

Figure 1 Flow chart describing the patient selection process

2. Descriptiv e study

2.1. Epidemiological characteristics

2.1.1. Frequency

Of 815 coronary bypass operations performed between January 2012 and December 2021 in the cardiothoracic surgery department at HMPIT, 77 patients had LV dysfunction, representing 10% of annual activity. The annual breakdown is shown in figure 2.

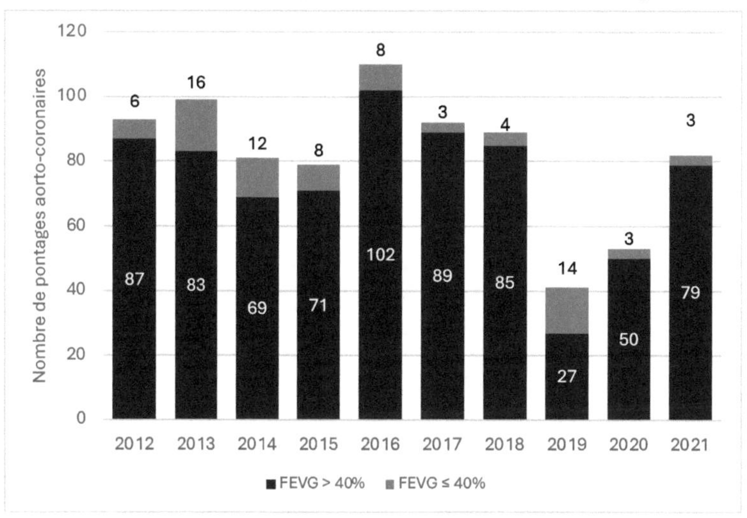

Figure 2 Annual distribution of patients undergoing coronary bypass surgery between 2012 and 2021

2.1.2. Type

In this study, 64 men (88%) and nine women (12%) were included.

2.1.3. Age

The average age of patients was 60.5± 7.5 years, with extremes ranging from 35 to 80 years . Table 2 compares average ages between the two genders.

Table 2 Average age of patients by gender

Age		Average	Standard deviation	Min	Max	p
Gender	Men	60,9	6,9	40	80	0.049
	Women	57,1	10,9	35	78	
Total		60,5	7,5	35	80	

Figure 3 summarizes the age and gender distribution of patients in our study.

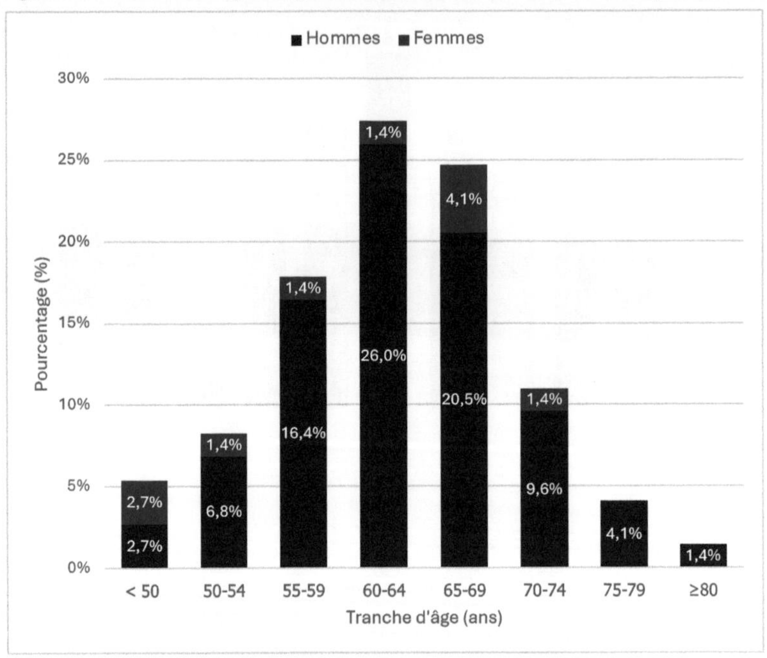

Figure 3 Patient distribution by age and gender

2.2. Cardiovascular risk factors

Cardiovascular risk factors were analyzed in the patients, as shown in Table 3 below:

Table 3: Distribution of cardiovascular risk factors by gender

Risk factor	Number of patients (%)	Men (%)	Women (%)	p
Smoking	50 (68)	49 (98)	1 (2)	$<10^{-3}$
Hypertension	34 (46)	29 (85)	5 (15)	0,725
Type 2 diabetes	40 (55)	32 (80)	8 (20)	0,035
Dyslipidemia	26 (36)	22 (85)	4 (15)	0,404
Familial coronary artery disease	1 (1)	1 (1)	0	-
Obesity	10 (14)	7 (70)	3 (30)	0,101

BMI was calculated retrospectively for 68 of the 73 patients in the study, i.e. 93% of the sample. The median BMI was 26 kg/m^2 with extremes of 14 and 36 kg/m^2 . Figure 4 shows the distribution of patients by body mass index.

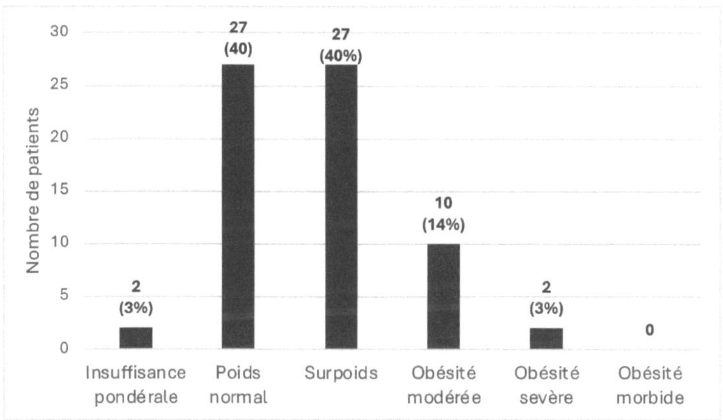

Figure 4 Distribution of patients by body mass index.

Every patient in the study had at least one cardiovascular risk factor, and 38 patients (52% of the sample) had three or more. Figure 5 shows the distribution of patients according to the number of associated cardiovascular risk factors.

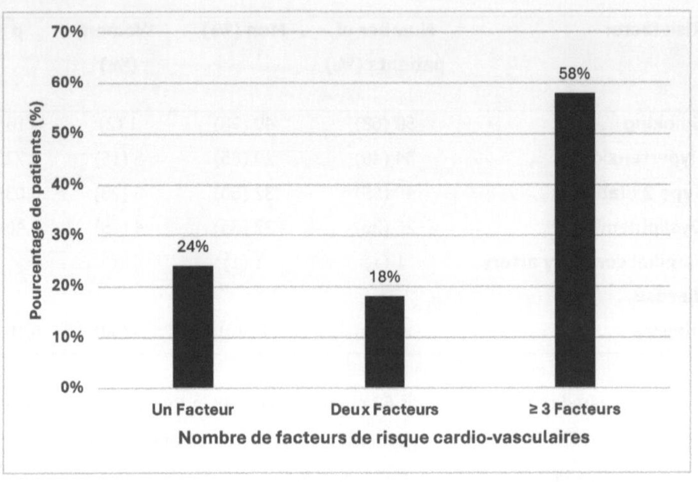

Figure 5 Distribution of patients by number of cardiovascular risk factors

2.3. History of coronary artery disease

2.3.1. Previous coronary syndromes

Of the 73 patients studied, 25 patients (34%) had had previous coronary events. The distribution was as follows:

- ✓ Three chronic coronary syndromes: one silent ischemia and two stable angina.
- ✓ Twelve STEMIs, including five semi-recent ones.
- ✓ Ten NSTEMIs at high risk of mortality.

2.3.2. History of transluminal angioplasty

Fifteen patients (21%) had a history of transluminal coronary angioplasty (TCA), with an average of 1.4 stents per patient. Figure 6 summarizes stent location.

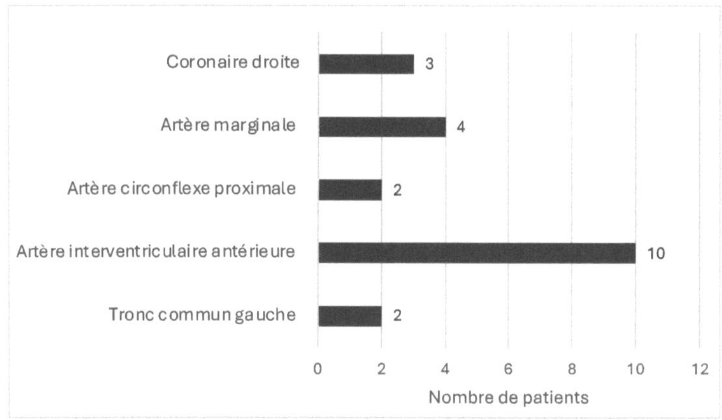

Figure 6 Angioplasty history

2.4. Other atheromatous localizations

2.4.1. Chronic obliterative arteriopathy of the lower limbs

Of the 10 patients (14%) with ACOMI, 80% were diabetic. Two underwent surgical revascularization (iliofemoral and femoro-popliteal bypass). One non-revascularized patient underwent leg amputation following dry gangrene.

2.4.2. Carotid atheroma n

Atheromatous carotid disease was identified in 15 patients (21%):

- ✓ Four had hemodynamically insignificant lesions on Doppler ultrasound of the internal carotid arteries.
- ✓ Eleven had internal carotid stenosis requiring further angioscanning. Tightness was confirmed in two of them. None underwent carotid endarterectomy combined with CABG.

2.4.3. Polyvascular disease

Three patients had polyvascular involvement, combining an internal carotid lesion and ACOMI.

2.5. History of strokes

Five patients (7%) had a history of stroke, four of which were constituted by ischemic stroke and one by transient ischemic attack. The probable etiologies of these strokes were :

- Significant carotid stenosis (n=1)
- Permanent atrial fibrillation (n=2)
- Intra-GV apical thrombus (n=1)
- Cryptogenic stroke (n=1).

2.6. Respiratory history

Eleven patients (15%) were being followed for COPD well balanced on treatment.

One patient had signs of chronic pleuropneumonia suggestive of pulmonary tuberculosis, but a negative Koch's bacillus test.

Two patients had COVID-19 infection without sequelae and underwent surgery six months after the virosis.

2.7. Clinical study

2.7.1. Circumstances of discovery

Figure 7 illustrates the circumstances in which coronary disease is discovered.

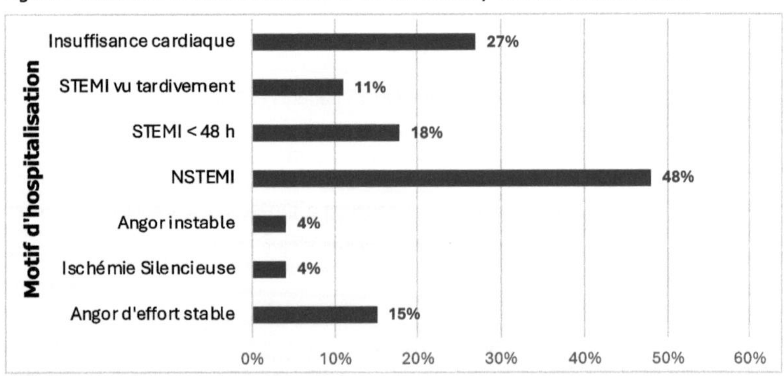

NSTEMI: Non-ST-segment elevation acute coronary syndrome

STEMI: persistent ST-segment elevation acute coronary syndrome

Figure 7 Distribution of patients according to circumstances of discovery

Six patients (2 NSTEMI and 4 STEMI) had benefited from a hybrid strategy involving percutaneous angioplasty of the culprit artery, before being referred to cardiac surgery for further myocardial revascularization by coronary artery bypass grafting.

Twenty patients (27%) had presented with signs of acute MI. Of these, one patient had dynamic ischemic MI, 15 were hospitalized for NSTEMI (43%), three patients for semi-recent STEMI, and one patient for acute MI flare-up revealing LV dysfunction due to silent ischemia.

2.7.2. Signs functional

In the month prior to myocardial revascularization surgery, 53 patients (72%) were paucisymptomatic and 20 patients (28%) were symptomatic, as shown in figure 8. No patient experienced syncope or lipothymia.

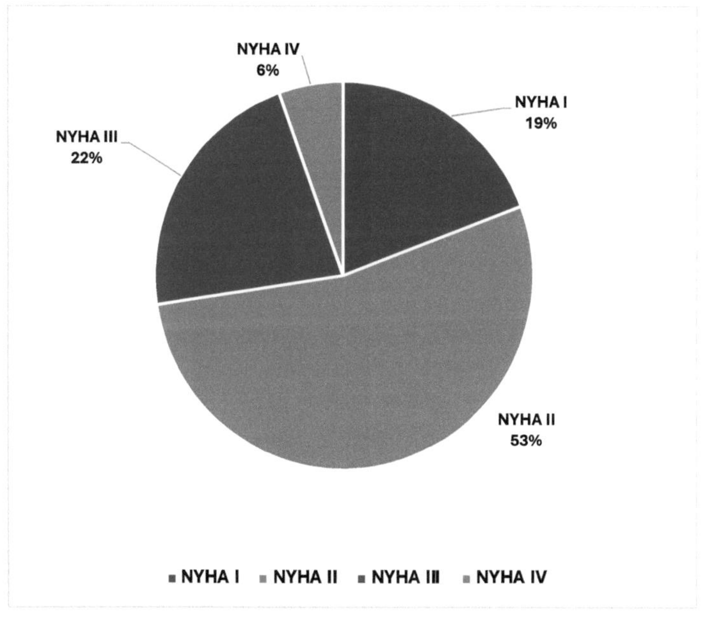

NYHA: New York Heart Association

Figure 8 Distribution of patients by degree of dyspnea

2.7.3. Examination physical

Fifty-one patients (70%) had a normal clinical examination at the time of surgery. Fifteen patients showed signs of left ventricular failure (LVF).

2.7.4. Electrocardiogram

Figure 9 shows the electrocardiogram (ECG) data, with sinus rhythm observed in 69 cases (94%).

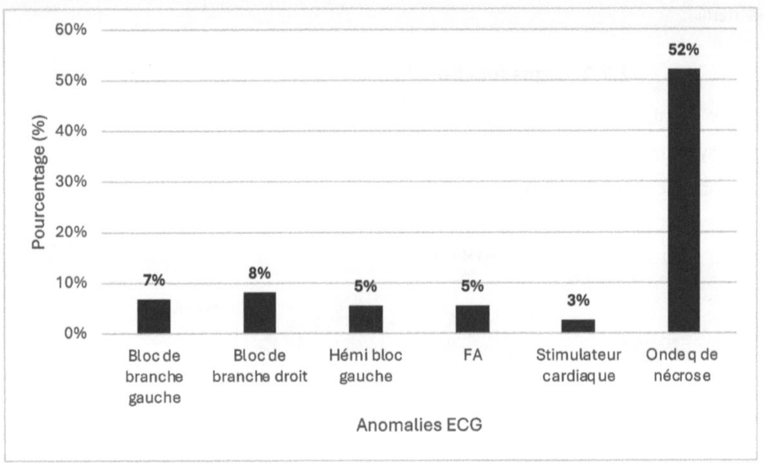

AF: Atrial Fibrillation

Figure 9 Distribution of different types of electrocardiographic abnormalities

One patient had a bi-fascicular block (a complete right bundle branch block with a left anterior hemiblock).

Two patients were fitted with dual-chamber pacemakers: the first to treat permanent complete atrioventricular block, and the second for second-degree sino-atrial block symptomatic of syncope. Eighteen patients had anterior necrosis sequelae and 19 patients inferior necrosis.

2.7.5. Preoperative biology

2.7.5.1. Blood count

Sixteen percent of patients, or twelve in total, had chronic anemia preoperatively. Table 4 summarizes the key values of preoperative haematological examinations for the study population.

Table 4: Preoperative biological parameters

Parameters	Mean ± SD Median (min-max)
Hemoglobin (g/dl)	13 ± 1.8 (7,4 - 15,7)
Hematocrit (%)	39,3 ± 4,9 (27,2 - 49)
Platelet count (10 /mm)^{33}	218 (103 - 544)
White blood cells (element/mm)^{3}	9070 (4700 - 16850)

2.7.5.2. Preoperative glycated hemoglobin

Among the subpopulation of diabetic patients, the mean HbA1c level was 8.9±2.2%, with extreme values ranging from 5.4% to 13.4%. Ninety-five percent of these patients had poorly controlled diabetes at the time of surgery.

2.7.5.3. Kidney function study

Mean creatinine clearance was 82.8 ± 31.6 ml/min. Thirty-five patients (47%) had chronic kidney disease, and seventeen patients (23%) had CKD, three of whom were on hemodialysis.

Among diabetic patients, 67% had at least one chronic kidney disease with decreased diuresis at the time of surgery, as shown in figure 10.

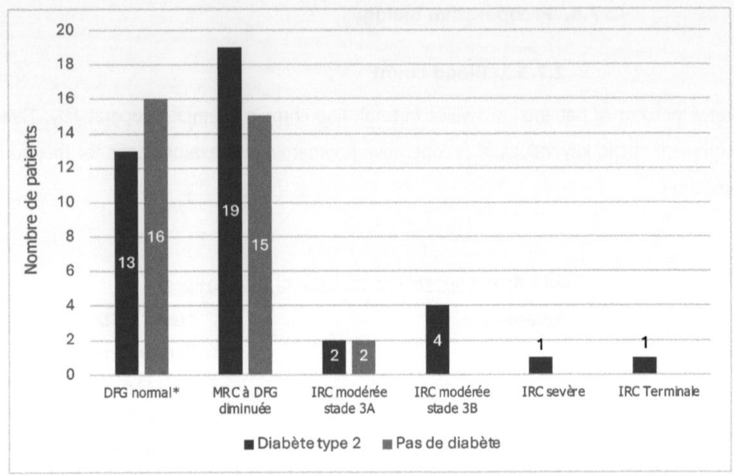

GFR: glomerular filtration rate, **CKD:** chronic kidney disease, **CKD:** chronic renal failure; * Renal function was considered normal in the absence of retrospective arguments in favor of CKD with preserved GFR.

Figure 10 Distribution of patients according to creatinine clearance and diabetes

2.7.5.4. Inflammatory assessment

The inflammatory profile of patients in this cohort was studied. Of the 67 patients for whom biological data were available, 49 (73%) had negative C-reactive protein (CRP) at the time of CAP. Of the 18 CRP-positive patients, five had CRP levels in excess of 50 mg/L.

2.7.6. Transthoracic echocardiography

2.7.6.1. Global left ventricular function

Mean LVEF was 37±3% with extremes between 25% and 40%. Among our patients, 36% had an LVEF ≤ 35% (Figure 11).

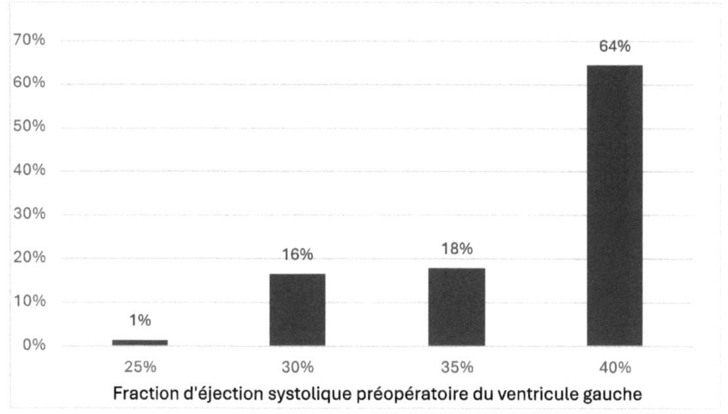

Figure 11 Distribution of patients according to preoperative LVEF

2.7.6.2. Disturbances in segment kinetics

Figure 12 details the distribution of segmental kinetic disorders on TTE.

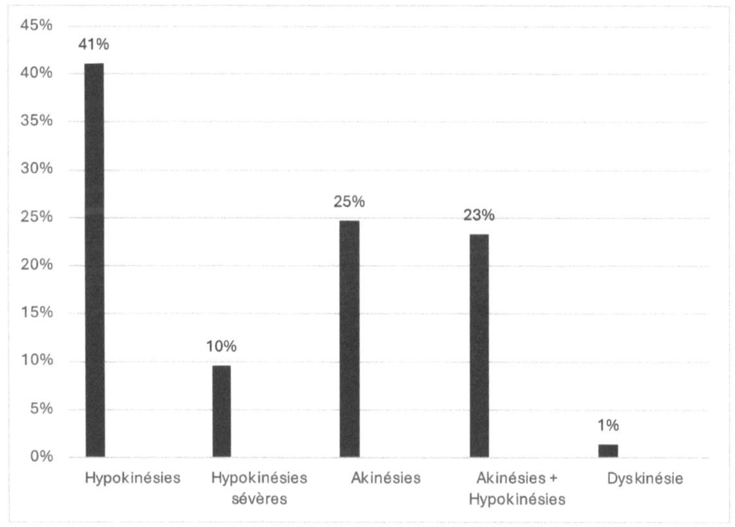

Figure 12 Segmental kinetics disorders

2.7.6.3. Other parameters of preoperative echocardiography

Parameters	n (%)	Mean ± SD (min-max)
Preoperative PAPS (mmHg)		37 ± 9 (24-65)
Left atrium surface area (cm)²		23 ± 5 (14-40)
Ischemic mitral insufficiency	2 (3)	
Increase in GWP	12 (17)	
Intra-VG thrombus	5 (7)	
VD dysfunction	1 (1)	

LV: Left ventricle, RV: Right ventricle, RVP: Right ventricle filling pressure

2.7.7. coronary angiography

2.7.7.1. Lesion status

Figure 13 summarizes the distribution of patients by lesion status, with a further distinction based on TCG involvement.

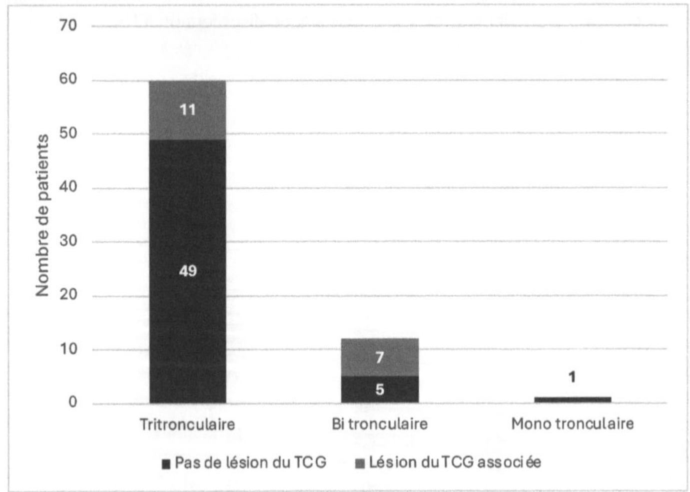

Figure 13 Distribution of patients according to lesion status and involvement of the left common trunk

2.7.7.2. Localization of coronary lesions

a. Damage to the anterior interventricular artery

The VIA was involved in 71 patients, i.e. 97% of cases. For the remaining 2 patients, the operative indication was for bi-truncular status in the face of distal TCG involvement, with no atheromatous extension to the VIA. The distribution of lesions according to segmentation of the VIA is illustrated in figure 14.

Of the 71 patients, 37 had involvement of the middle VIA (52%), 11 had distal involvement (15%), and seven (10%) had significant tandem lesions on all three segments.

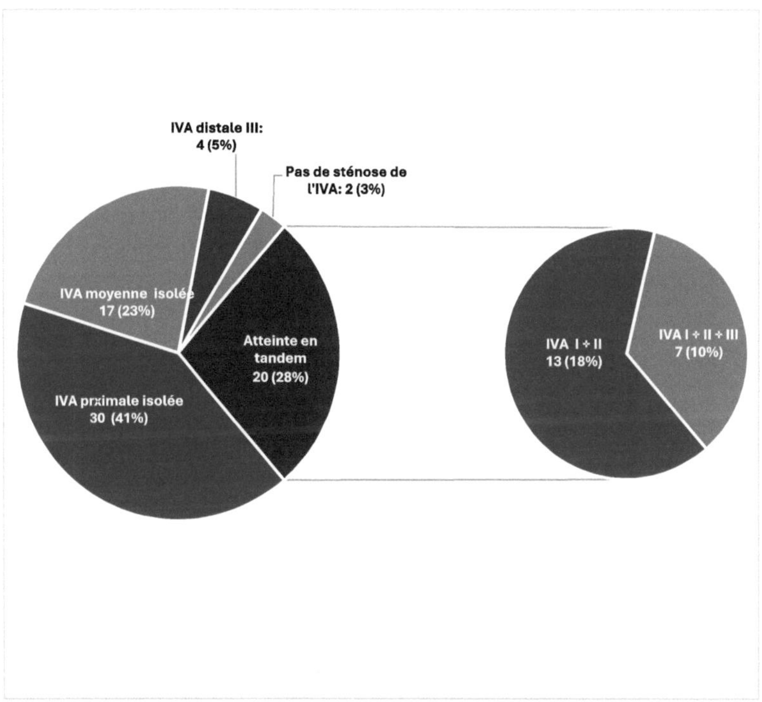

Figure 14 Distribution of atheromatous lesions on the IVA

b. Damage to the circumflex artery

The Cx artery was involved in sixty-seven patients, representing 92% of cases. Table 5 summarizes the location of these lesions.

Table 5: Angiographic characteristics of the circumflex artery

Lesion characteristics	n (%)
Lesions of the proximal circumflex artery - First marginal	50 (75)
Lesions of the distal circumflex artery	10 (15)
Multiple marginal lesions	7 (10)
Massive calcifications	2 (3)
Coronary network too small	10 (15)

Intraoperatively, bypass of the marginal arteries was rejected in 12 patients (18%). This decision was motivated either by the massive calcification observed in two patients, or by the very small caliber of the artery in the other ten.

c. Right coronary artery disease

Sixty-one patients (83.5%) had right coronary artery involvement. The distribution of lesions according to CD artery segmentation is illustrated in figure 15.

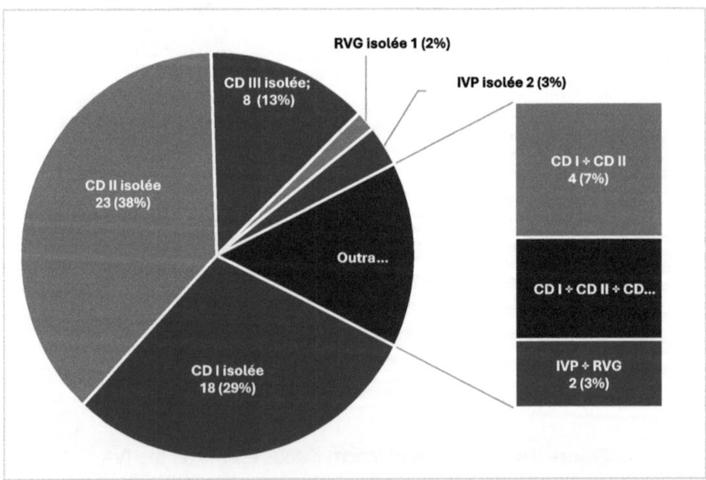

Figure 15 Distribution of lesions by segmentation of the right coronary artery

2.7.7.3. Stent restenosis

Of fifteen patients with a history of percutaneous angioplasty, five had experienced intra-stent restenosis, including two occlusive restenoses of the IVA artery. These restenoses had occurred on stents implanted as an emergency after an acute coronary syndrome in patients with type 2 diabetes.

2.7.7.4. Chronic total occlusions

Twenty-five patients (34%) had chronic total occlusion (CTO) of at least one coronary artery. Nine had double CTO and one patient had chronic total occlusions of all three coronary axes, as shown in figure 16.

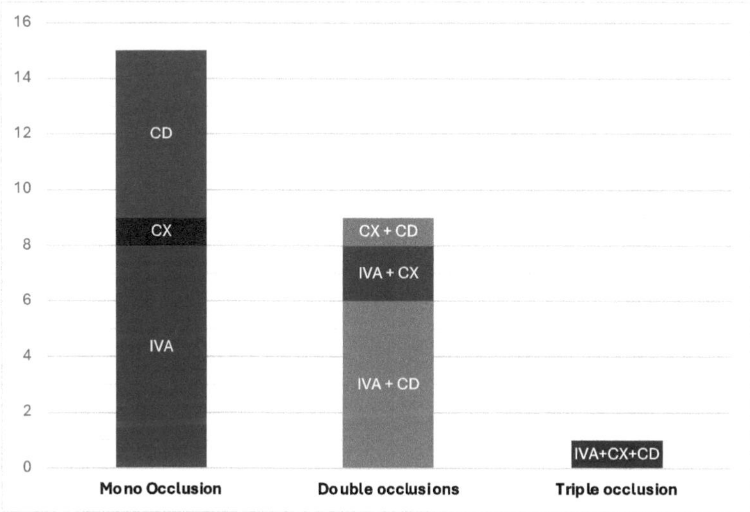

Figure 16 Distribution of chronic coronary occlusions

2.7.7.5. Coronary calcifications

Fourteen patients (19%) had calcified lesions. Of these, seven patients (10%) had calcifications affecting a single coronary axis, three patients (4%) had calcifications affecting two coronary axes, and four patients (6%) had calcifications affecting all coronary axes.

These calcifications were massive, circular and extended as far as the distal part of the IVA in one patient, the marginal artery in two patients (3%), and the CD artery in two others. In these four patients, intraoperative findings confirmed the impossibility of bypass surgery on calcified coronary arteries.

2.7.8. Study of myocardial viability

Preoperative, non-invasive myocardial viability testing was performed in nine patients, including seven severe akinesias and two severe hypokinesias, at resting TTE.
The types of viability tests requested are varied and are summarized in figure 17.

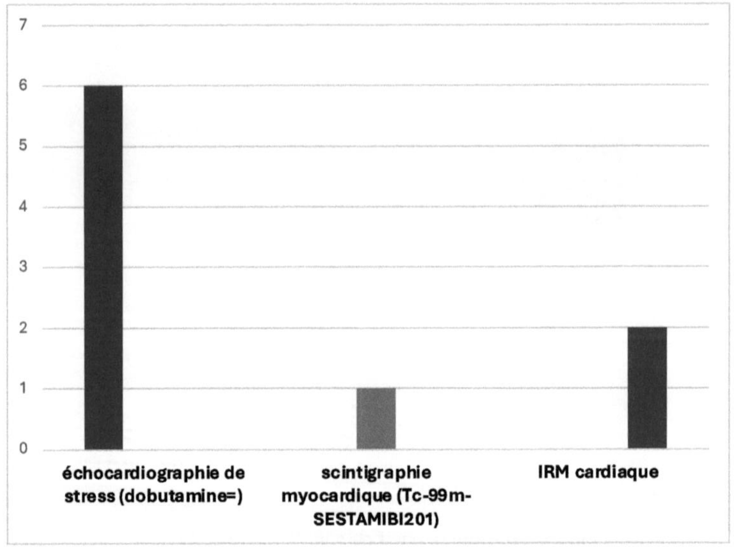

Figure 17 Types of viability tests requested

Table 6 shows the various clinical situations that have prompted the need for myocardial viability testing, and its impact on the patient's surgical management.

Table 6 Impact of myocardial viability tests on therapeutic strategy

	ATCD Coronary	Reason for hospitalization	FEVG (%)	Segmental kinetics	Coronary angiography	Type of viability test	Results	Coronary bypass surgery	Impact of viability testing
1	68 years old Men No medical history	Inferior STEMI (Thrombolysis)	30	Lower kinesia	Tritroncular lesions : ss calcified IVA I ss Cx-Mg ss CD	Stress echocardiography	No viability at the bottom	Coronary mono bypass surgery AMIG-IVA Mg: Bypass not feasible	Indication for coronary bypass surgery in tritruncal patients
2	53 years old Men NSTEMI ATL of the proximal IVA	NSTEMI	35	Anteroseptal Akinesia	Tritroncular lesions : RIS IVA I ss Proximal Cx CTO IVP	Cardiac MRI	Heart attack : Inferior-septal microvascular obstruction	Double PAC AMIG-IVA VSI-Marginal	Non-revascularization of a chronic non-viable IVP occlusion
3	62 years old Men No medical history	Stable angina	40	Severe hypokinesia of the apical cuff Restrictive ischemic MI	Tritroncular lesions : ss IVA ss 1ère Mg ss in Tandem CD I + II + III	Stress echocardiography	Viable myocardium Regression of MI grade on Dobutamine	AMIG-IVA VSI-Marginal CD: PAC not feasible	Ischemic MI probably reversible after revascularization
4	59 years old Men Semi-recent lower IDM	Stable angina	40	Apical cuff kinesis	Tritroncular lesions : CTO IVA I ss 1 Mgère ss CD II	Cardiac MRI	Viability of the anterior wall of the left ventricle	AMIG-IVA VSI-Mg VSI-CD	Surgical indication based on the presence of viability in the

	ATCD Coronary	Reason for hospitalization	FEVG (%)	Segmental kinetics	Coronary angiography	Type of viability test	Results	Coronary bypass surgery	Impact of viability testing
									IVA territory
5	68 years old Men Semi-recent IDM	NSTEMI	30	Akinesia of the entire septal wall	Bi-truncular lesions : ss very calcified IVA -Dg CD II CTO	Stress echocardiography	Presence of anterior and inferior wall viability	Monobypass AMIG - IVA Dg and CD deemed non-bridgeable	PAC indicated following viability test results
6	60 years old Men No medical history	NSTEMI	35	Hypokinesia of the anteroseptal wall Akinesia of the apical cuff and basal and medial segments of the lower wall	Tritroncular lesions : CTO of IVA II Ss Mg CD II CTO	Stress echocardiography	No viability at the bottom	AMIG-IVA AMID-Mg	Conversion from triple bypass to double CABG in the absence of viability in the right coronary territory
7	62 years old Men No medical history	NSTEMI	35	Lower dyskinesia Intra-VG thrombus	Tritroncular lesions : ss of distal TCG ss of IVA-Dg	Myocardial viability scintigraphy with Tc-99m-SESTAMIBI 201	Presence of Viability in the past Lack of viability in inferior and	AMIG - IVA AMID-Marginal Diagonal deemed hail	Conversion from triple bypass to double CABG in the absence

	ATCD Coronary	Reason for hospitalization	FEVG (%)	Segmental kinetics	Coronary angiography	Type of viability test	Results	Coronary bypass surgery	Impact of viability testing
					ss Proximal Cx CTO CD I		apical areas		of viability in the right coronary territory
8	54 years old Men No medical history	STEMI in lower (Thrombolysis)	35	Anterior, anteroseptal, inferoseptal kinesis	Single-truncular lesion: ss of bifurcation IVA-1ère diagonal	Stress echocardiography	Presence of basal and apical viability of the anteroseptal wall, anterior wall and inferoseptal wall Lack of viability limited to the anteroseptal wall (middle segment)	Single-deck AMIG-IVA Small diagonal intraoperatively	
9	65 years old Men No medical history	STEMI in lower Primary angioplasty of the right coronary artery	40	Akinesia of the basal and middle segments of the	Tritroncular lesions : ss of distal TCG ss IVA I - Dg, ss of Mg1,	Stress echocardiography	Presence of lower viability	AMIG-Diagonal, IVA VSI, Marginal, IVP	Coronary bypass of PVI retained following viability test results

ATCD Coronary	Reason for hospitalization	FEVG (%)	Segmental kinetics	Coronary angiography	Type of viability test	Results	Coronary bypass surgery	Impact of viability testing
			lower wall	IVP ss				

AMID: Right internal mammary artery, **AMIG:** Left internal mammary artery, **ATCD:** Past history, **ATL:** Transluminal angioplasty,

CD: right coronary artery, **CTO:** chronic total occlusion, **Cx:** circumflex artery, **Dg:** diagonal artery, **LVEF:** left ventricular ejection fraction, **MI:** mitral insufficiency, **MRI:** magnetic resonance imaging, **IVA:** anterior interventricular artery, **IVP:** posterior interventricular artery, **Mg:** Marginal artery, **CABG:** Coronary artery bypass graft**, RIS:** Intrastent restenosis, **RVG:** Left retroventricular artery, **SS:** Tight stenosis, **NSTMI:** Non-ST-segment elevation acute coronary syndrome, **STEMI:** ST-segment elevation acute coronary syndrome, **Tc:** Technetium, **TCG:** Left common coronary trunk, **LV:** Left ventricle, **VSI:** Long saphenous vein.

2.8. Medical treatment

All patients admitted with acute coronary syndrome had received anti-ischemic therapy prior to coronary angiography, and had been put on medical treatment prior to CABG. Figure 18 summarizes the different molecules prescribed for each therapeutic family.

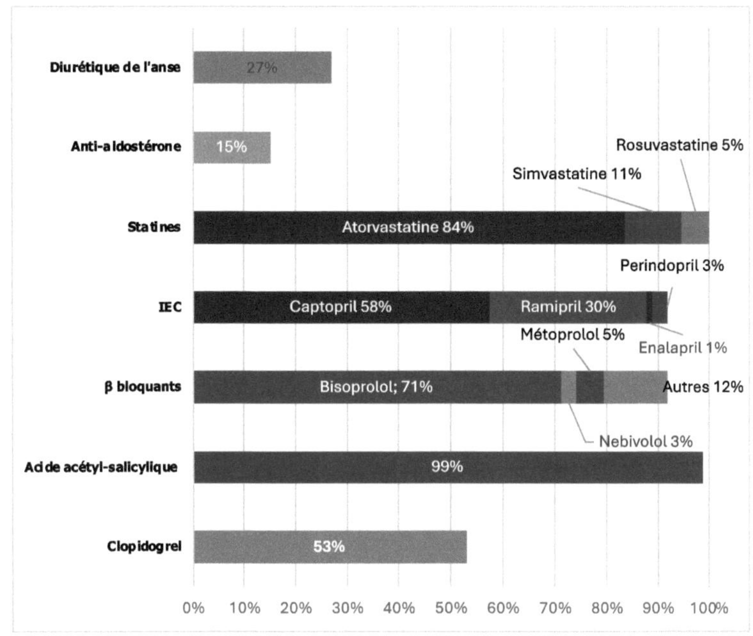

IEC: Enzyme-converting enzyme inhibitor

Figure 18 Different molecules prescribed before surgery

One patient had a known allergy to aspirin.

One patient required preoperative BCPIA circulatory support

Five patients (7%) received a prophylactic protocol of Levosimendan preoperatively.

2.9. Calculation of predictive scores for early mortality

2.9.1. Euroscore II

The mean for EUROSCORE II was 2.81±2.17%, with extreme values ranging from 1 to 11%.

Figure 19 summarizes the distribution of patients according to the degree of theoretical risk of 30-day mortality calculated by Euroscore II.

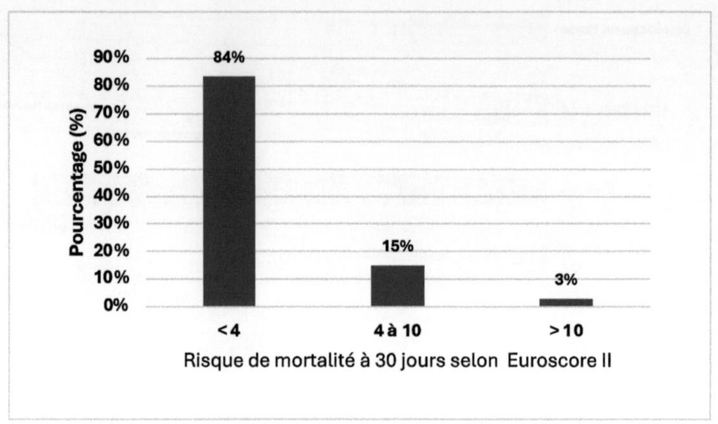

Figure 19 Distribution of patients by EUROSCORE II status

2.9.2. STS Risk-Score

Table 7 summarizes the postoperative risks assessed by the STS Risk-score 4.2.

Table 7 Prediction of various risks using the STS Risk-score 4.2

Estimated risk according to STS score 4.2	Average %	Standard deviation	Median %	Interquartile range	Min %	Max %
Mortality	1,30	1,07	0,88	0,90	0,42	6,69
Mortality	12,67	12,89	8,13	5,42	1,64	67,62

2.10. Coronary bypass surgery

All our patients underwent surgical myocardial revascularization under CEC. The approach was a median sternotomy.

2.10.1. Operating time s

Time to surgical myocardial revascularization varied significantly, with a median of 39 days (range 3 to 262 days) from coronary angiography. Only five percent of patients underwent surgery within 15 days of diagnosis, and 75% after one month. The six patients requiring perioperative BCPIA circulatory support were managed more quickly, with a median of 26 days (p=0.047).

The distribution of patients by time to surgery is shown in figure 20.

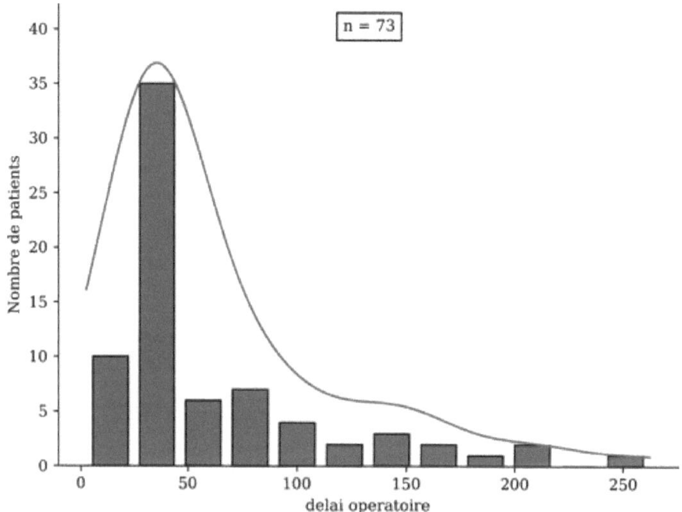

Figure 20 Distribution of patients according to operating time

2.10.2. Number of grafts and distal anastomoses

One hundred and ninety-two distal anastomoses were performed, representing an average of 2.6 ± 0.8 distal anastomoses per patient. Of these patients, 53% had at least one arterial anastomosis and 22% had exclusively arterial coronary bypass grafts. The distribution of patients according to the number of grafts used is detailed in figure 21.

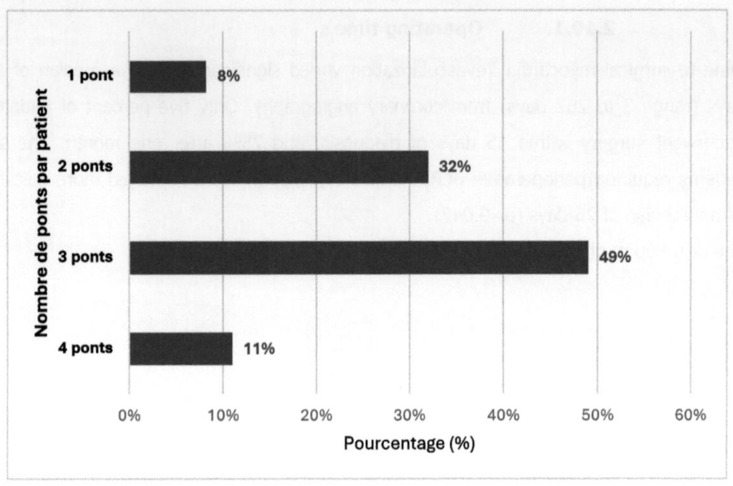

Figure 21 Distribution of patients by number of grafts

2.10.3. Types of grafts used

2.10.3.1. Left internal mammary artery

- ✓ Used as an arterial graft on the IVA in all patients.
- ✓ Sequential bridging of the IVA and diagonal in 9 cases (12%).

2.10.3.2. Right internal mammary artery

- ✓ For the 19 cases who had exclusively arterial coronary bypass through both mammary arteries (26%):
  - o Eight were pedicled, passing through the sinus of Theile (42%).
  - o Eleven were free graft, Y-anastomosed on AMIG, in 11 cases (58%).
- ✓ Used to revascularize a marginal or bisecting artery in 14 patients:
  - o Y rise in 9 patients.
  - o Pedicled in 5 patients.
- ✓ Sequentially anastomosed in two patients.

2.10.3.3. Long saphenous vein

- ✓ Used in 59 patients (81% of cases):
  - o Y on AMIG for a patient.
  - o As a single graft in 31 patients (42%).
  - o As multiple grafts (two or more) in 28 patients.
- ✓ A venous graft was sequentially anastomosed in three patients.

Figure 22 illustrates the distribution of coronary arteries revascularized by a venous graft.

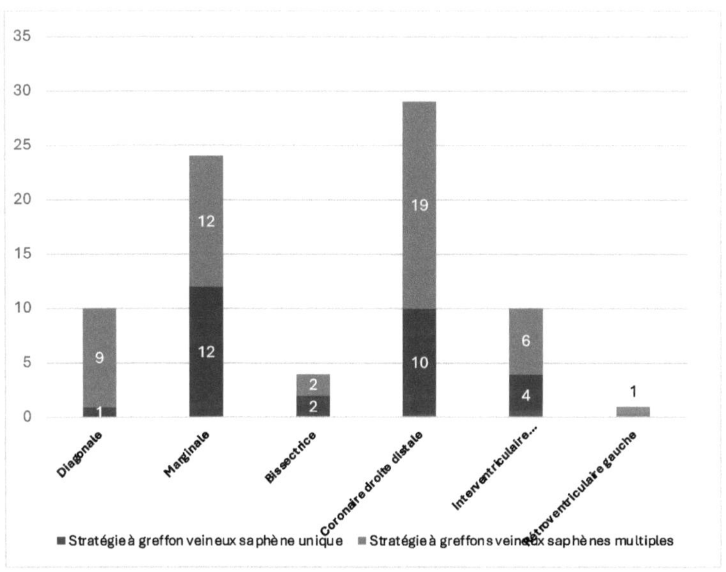

Figure 22 Distribution of coronary arteries revascularized with a venous graft

Figure 23 summarizes the different graft combinations used.

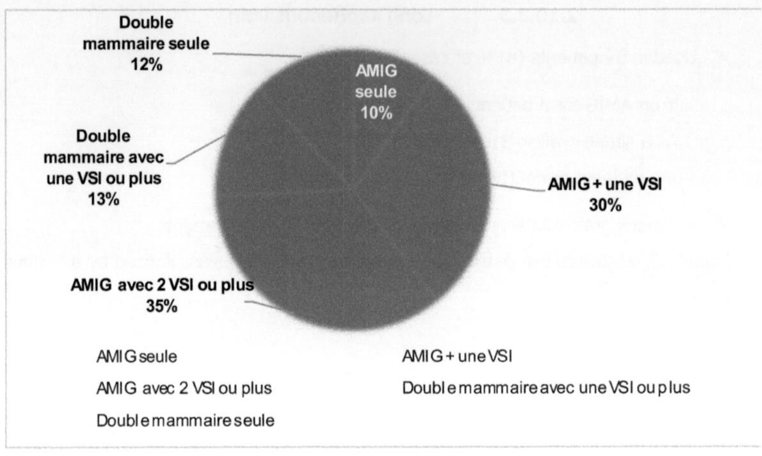

AMIG: Left internal mammary artery, **VSI:** Long saphenous vein

Figure 23 Different graft combinations used

2.10.4. Complete revascularization

Complete revascularization was achieved in 39 patients, or 53% (Figure 24).

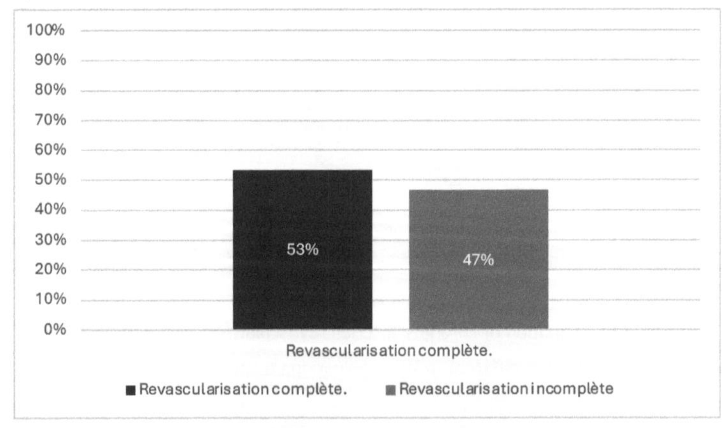

Figure 24 Index of myocardial revascularization

2.10.5. Study of extracorporeal circulation

Parameter	Mean ± SD (minutes)	Median	Min	Max
		(%)	(%)	(%)
CEC duration	124±46	119	37	350
Duration of aortic clamping	80±27	77	27	160
Circulatory assistance	34±3	7	284	

ECC: Extracorporeal Circulation

In 29 patients (41%), weaning from bypass was difficult, requiring administration of high doses of catecholamines for more than 24 hours.

BCPIA was initiated postoperatively in 15 patients (20%), while in four patients (5%), it was initiated intraoperatively and maintained after their weaning from CEC.

2.11. Morbi Early postoperative mortality

Immediate follow-up of patients was carried out in postoperative intensive care in the cardiovascular department, followed either by transfer to the cardiology department of the HMPIT, or a return home for patients with uncomplicated operative sequelae.

2.11.1. Length of stay in intensive care

Post-operative length of stay in the cardiovascular intensive care unit is summarized in figure 25.

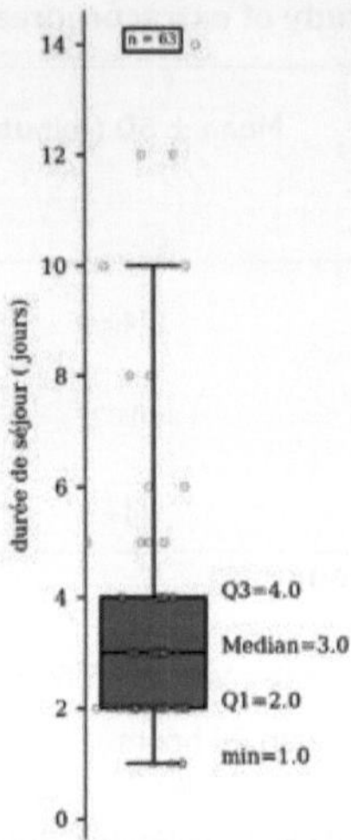

Figure 25 Postoperative length of stay in the cardiovascular unit

2.11.2. Duration of mechanical ventilation

The duration of mechanical ventilation was recorded in 68 cases (93%), with a median duration of 6±3 hours (2 to 240 hours). Mechanical ventilation lasted less than 12 hours in 72% of patients, less than 24 hours in 87%, and exceeded 48 hours in 11% of cases (Figure 26).

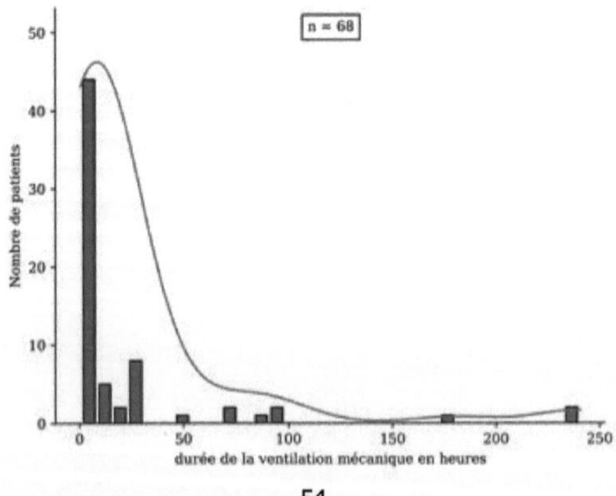

Figure 26 Duration of mechanical ventilation

2.11.3. Early postoperative hemoglobin and transfusions

The mean postoperative hemoglobin level was 9.5±1.4 g/dl, with extremes of 5.7 and 13.4 g/dl (figure 27).

Mean postoperative deglobulation was 3.6±1.6 g/dl, with extreme values ranging from 0.4 to 7.5 g/dl. With regard to transfusions, the median was 2 packed red blood cells (PRBCs) per patient, with an interquartile range of 2 PRBCs. Extreme values ranged from 0 to 6 RGCs.

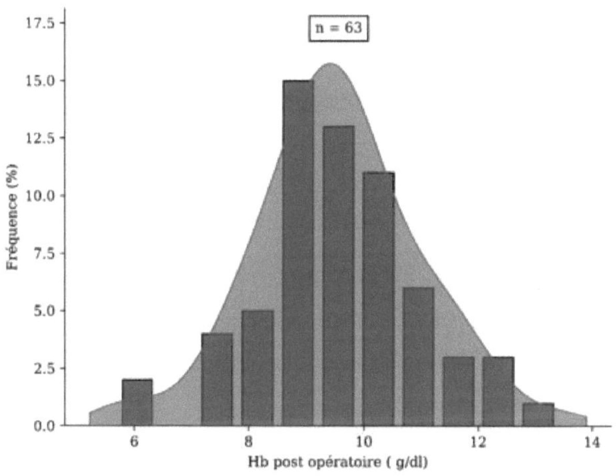

Hb: Hemoglobin

Figure 27 Distribution of postoperative hemoglobin levels

2.11.4. Major cardiovascular events early postoperative events

2.11.4.1. Early postoperative mortality

One patient died intraoperatively, and 15 patients (21%) within the first month postoperatively, bringing the early mortality rate to 22%.

The cause of intraoperative death was intractable intraoperative hemorrhage.

2.11.4.2. Early postoperative acute coronary syndromes

Twelve patients (17%) had early postoperative coronary events, including ten NSTEMIs and two STEMIs. Two patients died following NSTEMI complicated by cardiogenic shock. Postoperative coronary angiography was performed in three patients, revealing two VSI thromboses and a very tight anastomotic stenosis of the AMIG on the IVA .

2.11.4.3. Early postoperative strokes

Only one patient died following a massive stroke, diagnosed on postoperative day 2 and confirmed by a brain scan.

2.11.4.4. Postoperative low cardiac output syndrome

Of the 72 surviving patients, 44 (55%) showed signs of pulmonary congestion. Twenty-seven patients (37.5%) developed SBDC, 14 of whom required BCPIA.

Two patients required high doses of catecholamines for more than 48 hours and were treated with Levosimendan. Of the 27 patients who developed SBDC, 13 died.

2.11.4.1. Right ventricular failure

Eight patients (11%) developed deterioration of right ventricular longitudinal systolic function postoperatively.

2.11.5. Early postoperative major non-cardiovascular events

Table 8 summarizes the main early postoperative non-cardiovascular complications.

Table 8: Postoperative complications

Complications	n (%)
intrathoracic bleeding	1(1)
small to medium-sized pericardial effusions	13(18)
Pericardial tamponade	2(3)
Pulmonary embolism (PE)	1 (1)

Atrial fibrillation	3 (4)
Ventricular tachycardia	1 (1)
Complete atrioventricular block (pacemaker)	2 (3)
Infectious complications	25 (28)
acute renal failure	14(19)
Iatrogenic complications	2 (3)

Twenty-five patients (28%) developed a postoperative infectious syndrome, with the main sites of infection summarized in Figure 28. Six of the 25 infected patients died in hospital.

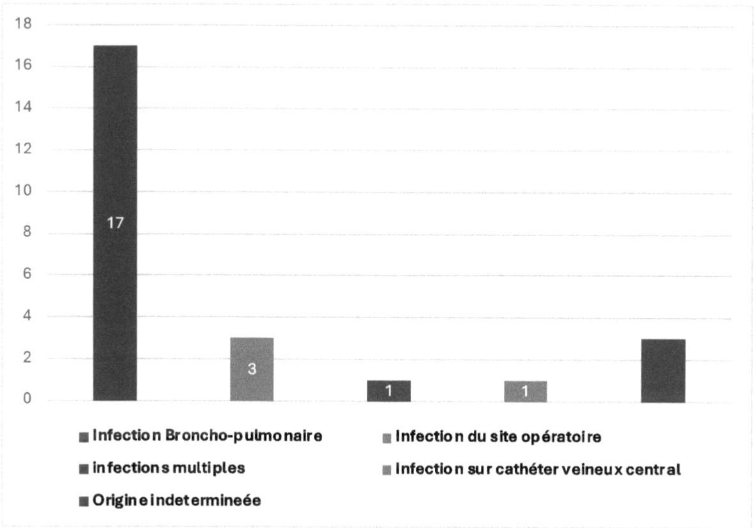

Figure 28 Localization of early postoperative infections

Two patients had a major iatrogenic complication, which was life-threatening:

- ✓ Acute ischemia of the left lower limb following iatrogenic dissection during placement of a BCPIA requiring emergency right and left aorto-femoral cross-bypass surgery, followed by left mid-thigh amputation.

- ✓ A case of rhabdomyolysis on statins

2.11.6. Early surgical revision

Eight patients (10%) required early revision surgery, the causes of which were :

- ✓ Two intrathoracic bleeds on postoperative day 1,
- ✓ A non-infectious sternal disunion operated on d9 postoperatively,
- ✓ Five early mediastinitis at D2, C4, 14, 17 and 19 days,

2.11.7. Evolution of LVEF in the early postoperative period

Post-operative LVEF could be found in 65 cases (89% of cases), either during the stay in the post-operative intensive care unit, or after transfer to the cardiology department.

The mean postoperative LVEF was 39.7 ± 7.6%, with a minimum value of 20% and a maximum value of 54%.

Early postoperative LVEF trends were distributed as follows:

Improved LVEF: 24 patients (37%)

Stable LVEF : 22 patients (34%)

Impaired LVEF : 19 patients (29%)

Sloping figure 29 illustrates the evolution of pre- and postoperative LVEF.

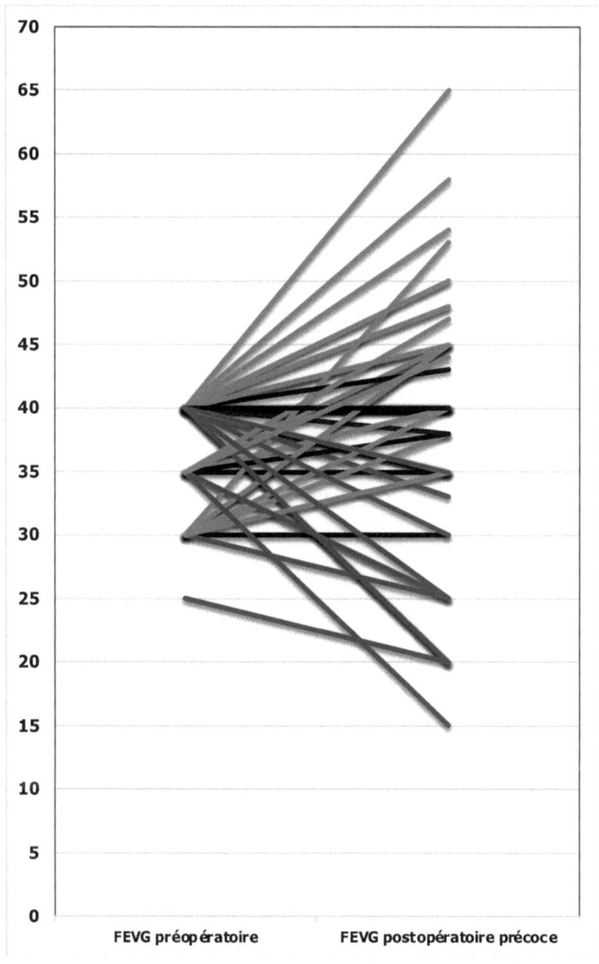

Figure 29 Evolution of LVEF in the early postoperative period

2.12. Patient follow-up

After one month, seven patients were lost to follow-up, and long-term follow-up involved 50 patients. The median follow-up was 95 months, with extremes ranging from one month to 134 months.

2.12.1. Changes in dyspnea during follow-up

Figure 30 illustrates the evolution of postoperative NYHA classification as a function of preoperative NYHA stage in the same patients.

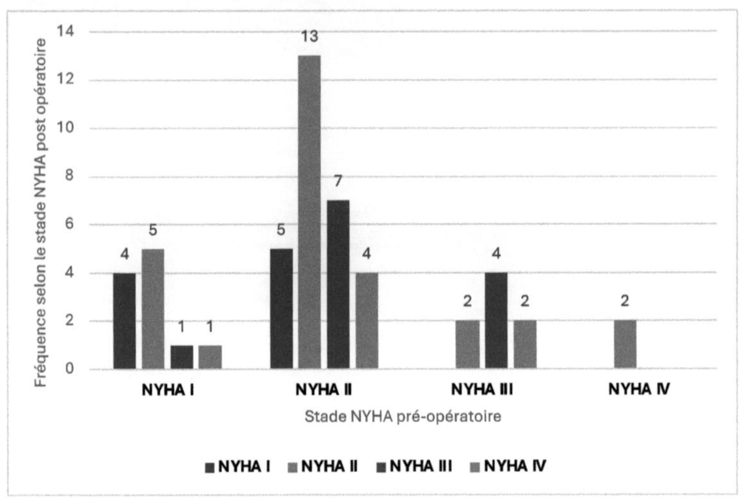

NYHA: New York Heart Association

Figure 30 Evolution of dyspnea postoperatively

2.12.2. Evolution of LVEF during follow-up

During follow-up, LVEF changes were distributed as follows:

Improved LVEF: 24 patients (48%)

Stable LVEF : 16 patients (32%)

Impaired LVEF : 10 patients (20%)

Figure 31 shows the evolution of LVEF during the different phases of the study.

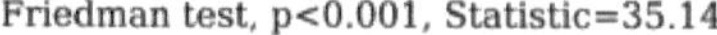

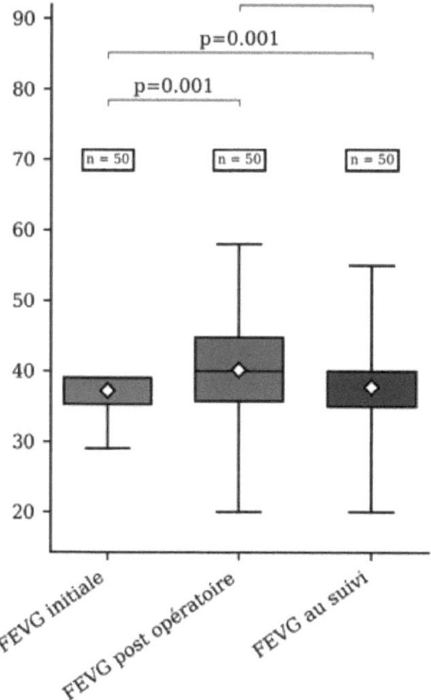

LVEF: Left ventricular ejection fraction

Figure 31 Evolution of LVEF during follow-up

2.13. Late postoperative major cardiovascular events

2.13.1. Late postoperative mortality:

The mortality rate beyond one month post-CAP was 40% (20 patients) for a median follow-up of eight years.

2.13.2. Acute coronary syndromes during follow-up :

In the population studied, nine patients developed ACS during their post-operative follow-up. Table 9 summarizes the coronary events, their delay and the course of action taken.

Table 9 Outpatient acute coronary syndromes

	Surgical gesture	Coronary syndrome	Coronary angiography	Driving
1	Triple PAC AMIG/IVA AMID/Mg VSI/IVP	Unstable angina after 20 months	AMID/Mg bypass occlusion	Marginal angioplasty
2	Double PAC AMIG/IVA VSI/CD	Unstable angina after 41 months	Permeable bridges Distal tight stenosis of a small Mg.	Medical treatment
3	Triple PAC AMIG/IVA AMID in Y on AMIG/Mg VSI/CD	Unstable angina after 81 months	Degenerated venous bridge	Right coronary angioplasty
4	Triple PAC AMIG/Dg-IVA VSI/Mg	Unstable angina after 22 months	Permeable bridges Intrastent restenosis of unbridged Mg	Marginal angioplasty
5	Dual PAC AMIG/IVA	Unstable angina after 75 months	Degenerated venous bridge Tight stenosis of the unbridged marginal Tight stenosis of the distal CD	Right marginal and coronary angioplasty
6	Dual PAC AMIG/IVA VSI/Mg	NSTEMI after 11 months	Tight stenosis of the proximal anastomosis of the VSI graft on the MG	ATC for VSI-Mg proximal anastomosis
7	Dual PAC AMIG /IVA VSI/Mg	NSTEMI after 32 years	Venous bridge over degenerated Mg Tight stenosis of CD III	Right marginal and coronary angioplasty
8	Triple PAC AMIG/IVA	NSTEMI after 36 months	Venous bridge over degenerated IVP	PVI angioplasty

	VSI/Mg VSI/IVP			
9	Triple PAC AMIG/IVA-DG VSI/Mg VSI/CD	NSTEMI after 42 months	Tight stenosis of the proximal anastomosis of the VSI / CD graft	ATC for VSI-CD proximal anastomosis

AMID: Right internal mammary artery, **AMIG:** Left internal mammary artery, **CD:** Right coronary artery, **Cx:** Circumflex artery, **Dg:** Diagonal artery, **IVP:** Posterior interventricular artery, **Mg:** Marginal artery, **NSTEMI:** Non-ST-segment elevation acute coronary syndrome**,** **CABG:** Coronary artery bypass graft, **RVG:** Left retroventricular artery, , **STEMI:** ST-segment elevation acute coronary syndrome **VSI:** Long saphenous vein.

2.13.3. Strokes during follow-up:

In our cohort, two patients presented a stroke of ischemic origin during follow-up, one at 4 months 19 days post CABG with no obvious cause and the other at 4 years 9 months post CABG in a patient with an apical thrombus treated with AVK.

Table 10 summarizes all MACCEs at the end of the study.

Table 10 Summary of major cardiovascular events

Events	**Major cardiovascular events**	
	Early	Late arrivals
Coronary	12	9
AVC	1	2
Deaths	16	20

STROKE : Cerebrovascular accident

3. Analytical study:

3.1. Predictors of early mortality

3.1.1. Study of qualitative parameters

In univariate analysis, the statistically significant factors predictive of early mortality are summarized in Table 11.

Table 11 Predictors of premature mortality

Risk factor	OR (IC95%)	p-value
Chronic renal failure	34 (7,4 ;155,7)	$<10^{-3}$
ACOMI	4,2 (1.1 ; 16,6)	0.044
NYHA III exertional dyspnea	4,6 (1,3 ; 16,1)	0,017
Preoperative abortion	4,7 (1,4 ; 16,0)	0,018
Tight TCG stenosis	5,1 (1,5 ; 16,9)	0,010
Multiple marginal lesions	6,7 (1,9 ; 23,3)	0,004
High-dose catecholamines over 24h	16,6 (3,3 ; 82,2)	$<10^{-3}$
Postoperative BCPIA	6,25 (1,7 ; 22,6)	0,007
Postoperative SBDC	15,5 (1,9 ; 126,5)	0,002
Myocardial infarction type 5	9,4 (2,5 ; 35,2)	$<10^{-3}$
Postoperative acute renal failure	6,3 (1,7 ; 22,6)	0,007
Post-operative infection	12,3 (3,3 ; 45,3)	$<10^{-3}$

ACOMI: Arteriopathie chronique des membres inférieurs, **BCPIA:** Ballon de contre pulsion intra aortique, **IVG:** Insuffisance ventriculaire gauche, **NYHA:** New-York Heart Association, **SBDC:** Syndrome de bas débit cardiaque, **TCG:** Tronc coronaire commun gauche

3.1.1.1. Study of quantitative parameters

Quantitative parameters predictive of early mortality are reported in table 12 (univariate analysis).

Table 12 Quantitative factors predictive of early mortality

Quantitative factors predictive of early mortality	Thresho ld value	OR (IC95%)	p-value

Euroscore II (%)	≥2,65	5,3 (1,56 ;18,8)	0,009
STS score (Mortality) (%)	≥1,24	5,2 (1,4 ;19,0)	0,01
Mechanical ventilation (H)	≥10	41,8(4,8 ;362,0)	$<10^{-3}$
Post-operative LVEF (%)	≤33	14,25 (5,5; 36,6)	$<10^{-3}$
Post-operative Hb (g/dl)	≤9,1	7,0 (1,32 ;37,1)	0,023

Hb: Hemoglobinemia, **LVEF:** Left ventricular ejection fraction

ROC curve analysis (Figure 32) detected two reliable markers predictive of early mortality:

- ✓ Duration of mechanical ventilation (Air under the curve = 0.823).
- ✓ Lower postoperative LVEF (Air under the curve = 0.979)

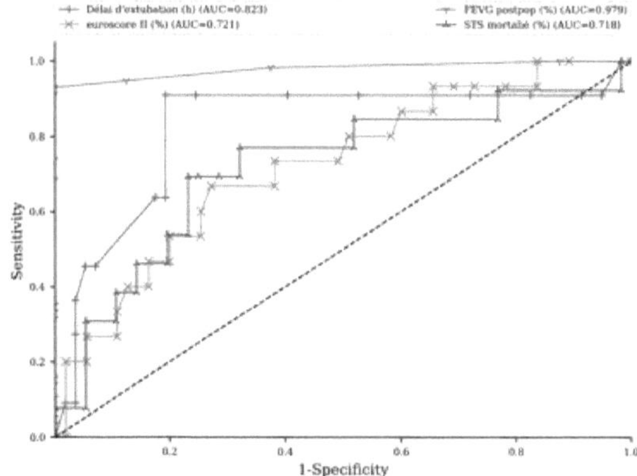

Figure 32 ROC curve analysis of quantitative risk factors for early post-operative mortality

3.1.1.1. Multivariate analysis :

Due to the limited number of late deaths, it was not possible to perform a multivariate analysis.

3.1. Predictors of major cardiovascular events in the early phase

Only CKD and postoperative infection were predictive of MACCE. Table 13 details the statistical study and results of the univariate study.

Table 13 Qualitative factors predictive of early major cardiovascular events

Risk factor	OR (IC95%)	p-value
Post-operative infection	4,96 (1,59 ; 15,41)	0,008
Chronic renal failure	7,58 (2,38 ; 24,21)	$<10^{-3}$

Quantitative parameters that had a statistically significant relationship with the occurrence of MACCE are reported in Table 14 (univariate analysis).

Table 14 Quantitative factors predictive of early major cardiovascular events

Risk factors	Threshold value	OR (IC95%)	p-value
Euroscore II (%)	≥3,18	5,24 (1,6 ;16,8)	0,014
STS score (Mortality) (%)	≥0,93	3,63 (1,3 ;10,3)	0,027
Mechanical ventilation (H)	≥9	6,2 (2,0 ;19,5)	0,007
Post-operative LVEF (%)	≤33	12,3 (3,0 ;50,0)	$<10^{-3}$

LVEF: Left ventricular ejection fraction, **MACCE:** Major cardiovascular events

ROC curve analysis failed to detect a reliable marker predictive of early MACCE (Figure 33).

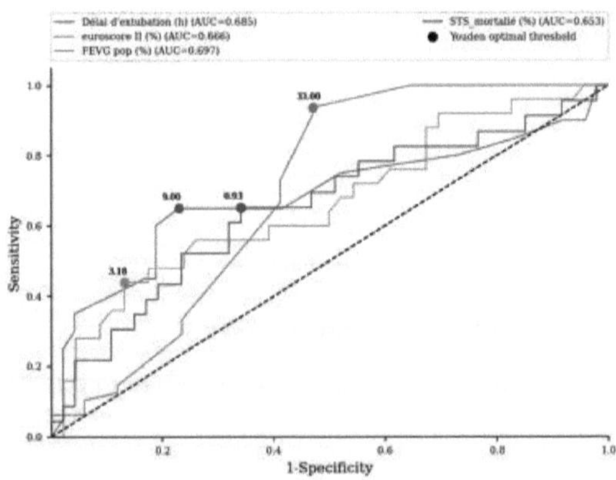

Figure 33 ROC curve analysis for quantitative risk factors for early major cardiovascular events

3.1. Predictors of early LVEF impairment

Risk factors for early post-operative LVEF impairment are summarized in Table 15.

Table 15 Predictors of postoperative LVEF decline

Risk factor	OR (IC95%)	p-value
Anteroseptal hypo/Akinesia	8,9 (1,9 ; 44,1)	0,003
Incomplete revascularization	6,5 (1,6 ; 26,1)	0,007
Tandem involvement of the VIA	4.05 (1,2 ; 13,6)	0,027
Distal Cx lesion	4,5 (1,1 ; 18,5)	0,027
Post-operative infection	12,6 (3,0 ; 53,1)	<0,001

IVA: Anterior interventricular, **Cx:** Circumflex artery

There was no statistically significant relationship between LVEF and postoperative right ventricular longitudinal systolic function (p = 0.79), nor with the presence of tandem CD lesions (p = 0.658).

Compared to the group of patients with unchanged or improved postoperative LVEF (Control Group), the group with worsening ejection fraction required more intensive resuscitation and had greater morbidity :

- ✓ post-operative intra-aortic BCPIA (OR = 6.0 (1.5; 23.9); p = 0.014).
- ✓ Catecholamines >24 hours (OR = 5.7 (1.6; 19.8); p = 0.006).
- ✓ High doses of loop diuretics (OR = 4.1 (1.2; 13.6); p = 0.027).
- ✓ Postoperative acute renal failure (OR = 10.1 (2.38; 42.4); p=0.002).
- ✓ SBDC postoperatively (OR = 8.9 (1.8; 44.1); p=0.003).
- ✓ Median length of stay in intensive care was four days for the group with impaired LVEF versus two for the control group (p= 0.038).
- ✓ Duration of mechanical ventilation was 24 hours for the group with impaired LVEF versus seven hours for the control group (p=0.031).

CEC time, aortic clamping time and cardiac assistance time were comparable in both groups, with respective p values of 0.155, 0.1 and 0.823.

3.1. Predictors of incomplete revascularization

Predictive factors of incomplete revascularization in univariate analysis:

Presence of coronary calcification (OR = 3.8 (1.1; 12.8); p=0.035)

The presence of tandem lesions on the VIA (OR = 4.2 (1.3; 13.2); p=0.035)

3.1. Predictive factors for postoperative low cardiac output syndrome :

Predictive factors for the occurrence of postoperative SBDC were:

- Chronic renal failure (OR = 3.43 (1.15; 10.21); p=0.031).
- LVEF ≤ 35% early post-op (OR = 7.97 (2.52; 25.24); p<0.001).
- Preoperative myocardial infarction (OR = 7.97 (2.52; 25.24); p<0.001).

3.2. Predictive factors for postoperative infections

In univariate analysis, factors predictive of the occurrence of postoperative infection were:

✓ Qualitative factors :

- History of dialysis (p = 0.039).
- Chronic obliterative arteritis of the lower limbs (OR = 6.9 (1.6; 29.1); p = 0.012).
- Significant internal carotid stenosis (OR = 4.2 (1.1; 16.1); p = 0.041).
- Post-operative acute renal failure (OR = 7.17 (1.9 ; 26.3); p=0.003).

✓ Quantitative factors :

- Risk of surgical site infection estimated ≥ 26% by online STS score calculator (OR = 4.9 (1.7; 14.5); p=0.005).
- BMI ≥ 25 kg/m^2 (OR= 3.34 (1.5; 5.2); p<10).$^{-3}$
- CEC time greater than 138 minutes (OR = 3.45 (1.2; 9.7); p=0.021).
- Aortic clamping time > 120 minutes (OR = 5.6 (1.0; 31.5); p=0.045).

There was no statistically significant relationship with these factors:

- Type 2 diabetes (p = 0.804)
- CRP preoperatively (p = 0.845).
- Preoperative ferritinemia (p = 0.246).
- Euroscore II (p = 0.809).
- STS score Morbi-mortality (p = 0.349).

This complication prolonged the duration of mechanical ventilation beyond 6 hours (OR = 4.8 (1.0; 23.4); p=0.041) and the length of stay in the cardiovascular intensive care unit to 5 days or more (OR = 6.4 (1.7; 24.4); p=0.007).

3.1. Predictors of acute renal failure

Parameters with a statistically significant relationship with postoperative impairment of Renal Function were:

- ✓ Qualitative parameters :
  - Acute postoperative CI (OR = 15.5 (1.9; 126.5); p = 0.002).
  - Postoperative infection (OR = 7.2 (1.9; 26.3); p = 0.003).
- ✓ Quantitative parameters :
  - Postoperative LVEF <38% (OR=3 (1.8; 5.1); p = 0.001).
  - Duration of mechanical ventilation >48h (OR=35.3 (4.7; 256.5); p<10).$^{-3}$
  - STS score Morbi-mortality < 7.66% (OR=1.9 (1.4, 2.63); p = 0.017).
  - BMI>26 kg/m2 (OR=1.8 (1.07, 3.0); p<10-3).

ROC curve analysis detected only one reliable marker predictive of acute renal failure: prolonged mechanical ventilation beyond 48 hours, with an area under the curve of 0.876 (as shown in figure 34).

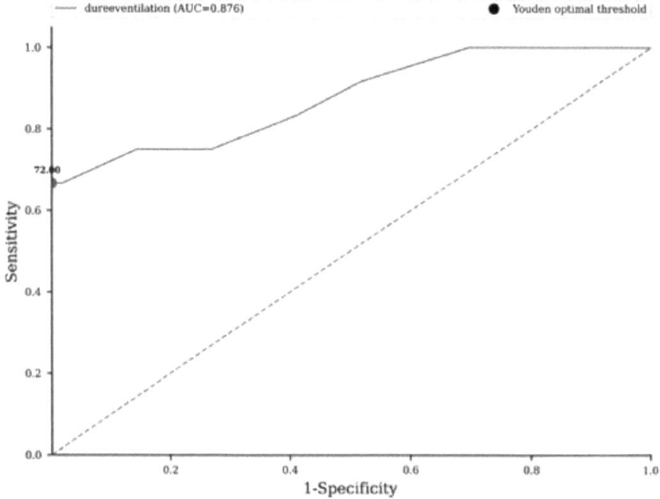

Figure 34 ROC curve analysis for prolonged mechanical ventilation as a predictive marker for acute renal failure

Beyond 24 hours of ventilation, a sensitivity of 66.7% and a specificity of 98.2% were obtained, with a positive predictive value (PPV) of 88.9% and a negative predictive value (NPV) of 93.2%. When the duration of mechanical ventilation reached 48 hours, the sensitivity and specificity values increased to 66.7% and 100% respectively, and the PPV and NPV rose to 100% and 93.3%.

3.2. Predictive factors for prolonged mechanical ventilation

Independent predictors of duration of mechanical ventilation in multivariate analysis were:

- ✓ SBDC with postoperative mechanical circulatory support (β=37.28, p=0.0023);
- ✓ Postoperative infection (β=30.82, p= 0.0216);
- ✓ Postoperative impairment of LVEF (β=46.54, p= 0.0181).

3.1. Predictors of late mortality

Factors predictive of late mortality, in univariate analysis, are summarized in Table 16.

Table 16 Risk factors for late mortality

Risk factor	Threshold value	**Univariate analysis**	
		OR (IC95%)	**p-value**
Kinetic anomalies in the Anteroseptal region		5,4 (1,6 ; 18,7)	0,009
Emergency surgery (on clopidogrel)		3,7 (1,1 ; 12,2)	0,043
Acute or late mediastinitis		-	0,021
LVEF improvement during follow-up		0,1 (0,03-0,47)	0,002
Preoperative leukocytes (10 /mm)^{33}	≥8,7	5,2 (1,4 ;18,6)	0,01
HbA1c (%)	≥9	30,0 (2,14 ;421,1)	0,009
LVEF during follow-up (%)	≤-5	9,5 (1,11 ;81,5)	0,03

ΔLVEF during follow-up (%)	≥+5	0,1 (0,03 ;0,47)	0,03

HbA1c: glycated haemoglobin, **LVEF:** left ventricular ejection fraction **ΔLVEF:** LVEF during follow-up - preoperative LVEF

It should be noted that neither the Euroscore II nor the STS score proved to be statistically significant predictors of late mortality, with p-values of 0.095 and 0.120 respectively. Analysis of the ROC curves (Figure 35) revealed only one reliable quantitative marker for predicting late mortality: preoperative HbA1c, with an area under the curve of 0.802.

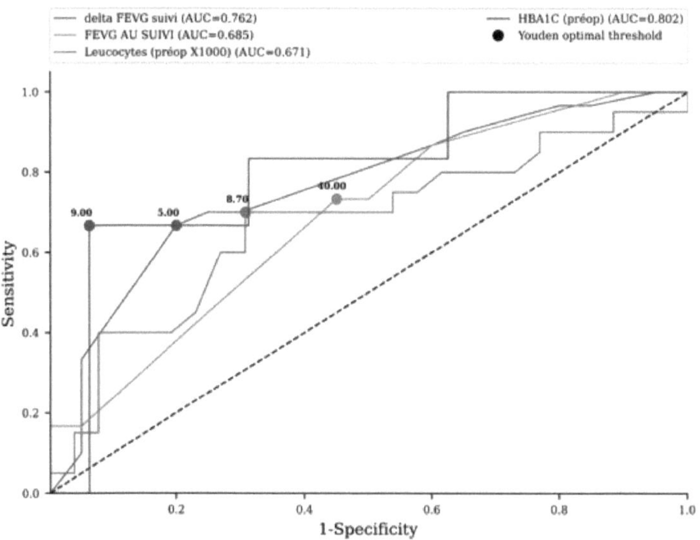

AUC: Area under the curve, **LVEF:** Left ventricular outflow fraction,

Figure 35 ROC curves for quantitative risk factors for late postoperative mortality

As shown in figure 36, even long-term mortality was higher among poorly balanced diabetics at the time of CAP.

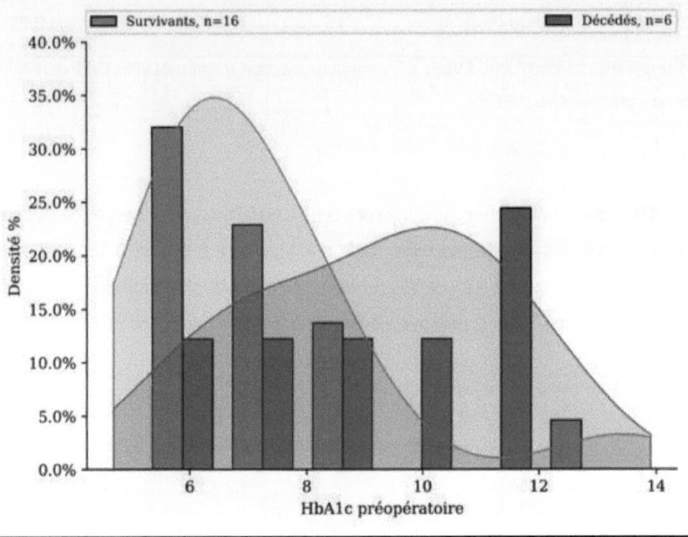

HbA1c: glycated hemoglobin

Figure 36 Distribution of late deaths according to preoperative glycated hemoglobin in diabetics

A multivariate analysis could not be performed due to the low number of events.

3.2. Predictors of late postoperative major cardiovascular events

Table 17 summarizes the predictive factors for late MACCE (univariate analysis).

Table 17 Qualitative risk factors for late major cardiovascular events

Risk factors	Univariate analysis	
	OR (IC95%)	**p-value**
Preoperative acute IC	8,5 (1,1 ; 69,6)	0,027
Chronic renal failure	7,5 (2,4 ; 24,2)	$<10^{-3}$
Extreme emergency surgery on clopidogrel	4,5 (1,5 ; 13,7)	0,027

Post-operative infection	5,6 (1,1 ; 27,3)	0,036
Disturbances in anteroseptal segmental kinetics	4,7 (1,4 ; 15,0)	0,009
LVEF improvement during follow-up	**0,2 (0,09 ; 0,8)**	0,049

LVEF: Left ventricular ejection fraction, **HF:** Heart failure, **MACCE:** Major cardiovascular events

3.3. Predictors of overall mortality

3.3.1. Study of qualitative parameters

Statistically significant risk factors for overall mortality are summarized in Table 18 (Univariate analysis).

Table 18 Qualitative predictors of overall mortality

Risk factor	Univariate analysis	
	OR (IC95%)	**p-value**
Chronic renal failure	34 (7,42- 155,75)	**$<10^{-3}$**
Preoperative abortion	3,67 (1,04- 12,86)	**0,049**
Segmental kinetic anomalies in the Anteroseptal region	2,91 (1,05 - 8,09)	**0,048**
Anomalies in anterior segment kinetics	4,57 (1,57- 13,30)	**0,005**
Emergency surgery (on Clopidogrel)	3,14 (1,14 - 8,65)	**0,029**
Catecholamines beyond 24h	5,81 (1,96- 17,21)	**0,001**
Postoperative BCPIA	4,50 (1,13- 17,87)	**0,038**
Degradation of renal function	7,30 (1,48- 36,01)	**0,013**
Post-operative infection	6,00 (1,52- 23,64)	**0,010**

BCPIA: Ballon de contre pulsion intra Aortique, **IVG:** Insuffisance ventriculaire gauche

Improvement in LVEF during follow-up was the only statistically significant protective factor reducing overall mortality (OR=0.1 (0.1; 0.5); p=0.002).

3.3.2. Study of quantitative parameters

Quantitative parameters that had a statistically significant relationship with overall mortality are reported in table 19 (univariate analysis).

Table 19 Quantitative risk factors for overall mortality

Risk factors	Threshold value	OR (IC95%)	p-value
Euroscore II (%)	≥1,88	5,73 (1,9 ;16,9)	0,003
STS score (Mortality) (%)	≥0,88	4,6 (1,6 ;13,48)	0,008
Mechanical ventilation (H)	≥10	6,9 (1,95 ;24,6)	0,004
Immediate postoperative LVEF (%)	<40	5,0 (1,63 ;15,82)	0,009
Preoperative Hb (g/dl)	<12,4	4,9 (1,4 ;17,2)	0,013
Post-operative Hb (g/dl)	<9,2	5,2 (1,7 ;16,5)	0,007
LVEF during follow-up (%)	<35	4,3 (1,1 ;17,2)	0,04

LVEF: Left ventricular ejection fraction, **Hb:** Hemoglobinemia

Analysis of the ROC curves did not reveal any reliable predictor of overall mortality. Indeed, for all statistically significant parameters, the area under the curve never exceeded 0.75 (Figure 37).

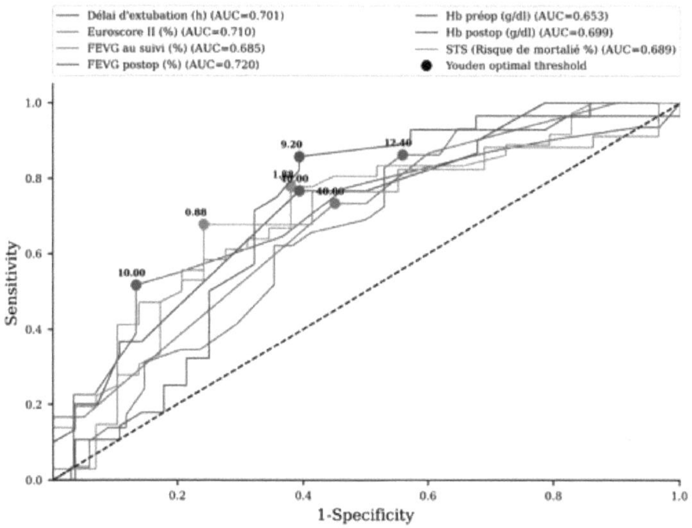

Figure 37 ROC curve analysis of predictors of overall mortality

3.3.3. Multivariate analysis

In multivariate analysis, the independent factors predictive of mortality were :

- ✓ The presence of segmental kinetic disorders in the anterior or anteroseptal territory (OR=4.21; 95% CI (1; 15.77); p= 0.033),
- ✓ Emergency surgery following ACS (on clopidogrel) (OR=1.1; 95% CI (1.45; 17.92); p= 0.011),
- ✓ The use of catecholamines for a duration ≥ 24 hours in the immediate postoperative period (OR=9.79; 95% CI (2.61; 36.75); p= 0.0007)

4. Survival analysis:

4.1. Overall survival analysis

The median follow-up in our study was 8 years, with a minimum of one year and a maximum of 11 years. Kaplan-Meier survival analysis (Figure 38) revealed that survival in our cohort was 68.5% at 2 years, with a 95%

confidence interval ranging from 56.5% to 77.8%. At 5 years, the survival rate was 57.9%, with a 95% CI between 45.5% and 68.5%.

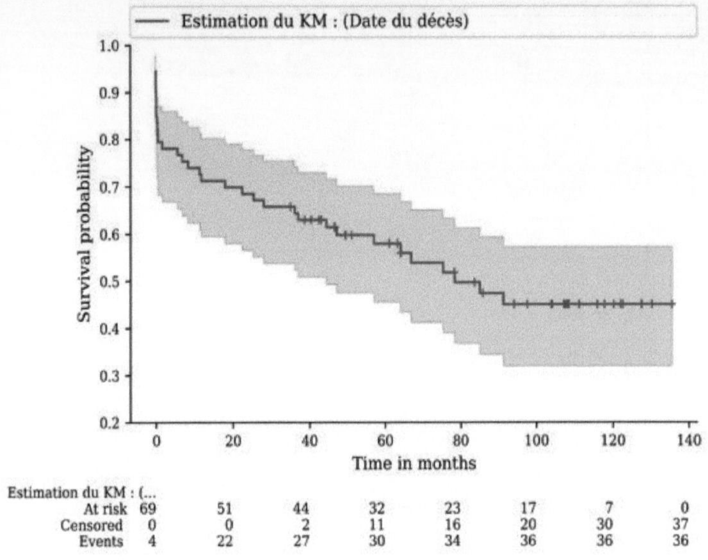

Figure 38 Kaplan-Meier survival analysis (Event=Death)

4.2. Analysis of survival as a function of postoperative changes in left ventricular ejection fraction

4.2.1. According to early postoperative LVEF

Early postoperative LVEF was stratified into three groups: worsened, unchanged and improved. Survival curves showed no statistically significant difference between these groups (Log Rank = 0.06), as illustrated in Figure 39.

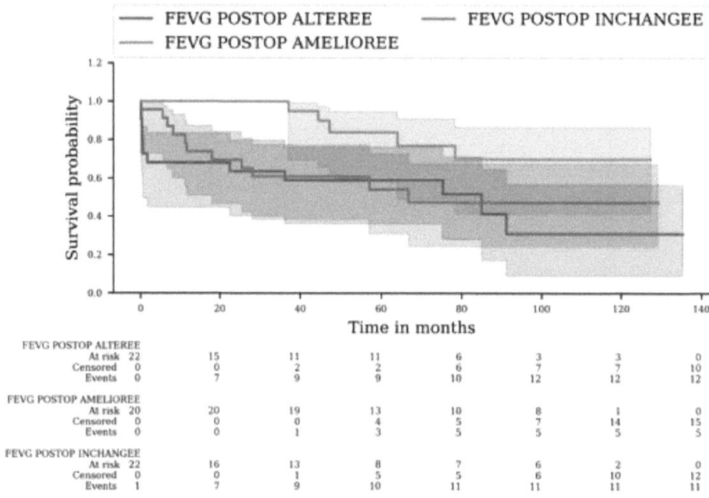

Post-op LVEF: Post-operative left ventricular ejection fraction

Figure 39 Analysis of survival according to early postoperative evolution of left ventricular ejection fraction

However, bivariate analysis (Figure 40) revealed a statistically significant difference in survival distributions between the degraded and improved postoperative LVEF groups (Log Rank < 10^{-3}).

At 24 months, survival rates were 46.7% (95% CI (28.4; 63.0)) and 100%, and at 5 years, 43.3% (95% CI (25.6; 59.9)) and 84.0% (95% CI (57.9; 94.6)), respectively.

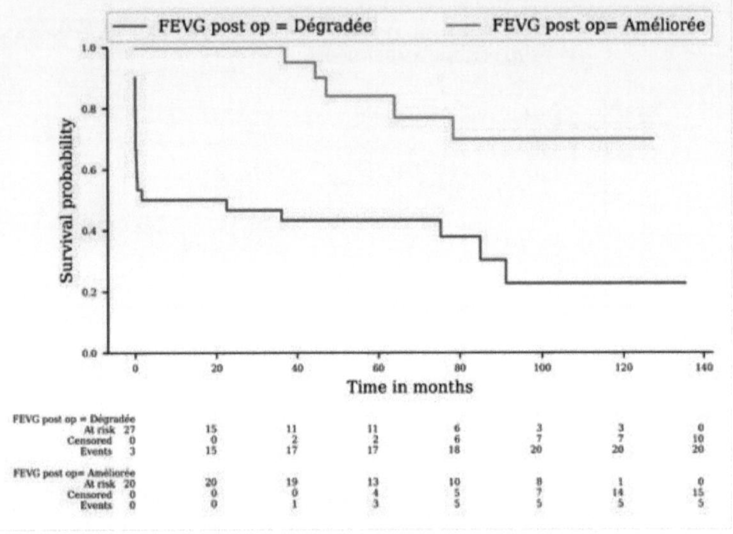

Post-op LVEF: Post-operative left ventricular ejection fraction

Figure 40 Binary analysis of survival according to early postoperative evolution of left ventricular ejection fraction (Impaired Vs Improved)

In multivariate Cox regression, early LVEF impairment was associated with a four-fold higher risk of death, compared with LVEF improvement (HR=3.62, 95% CI (1.4 - 9.37), p = 0.007).

4.2.2. Based on LVEF during follow-up:

No significant difference was observed between the survival distributions of the impaired and unimpaired LVEF groups. However, a significant difference was noted with the improved LVEF group (Log Rank =0.014), as shown in figure 41.

At 24 months, survival was 70.0% with 95% CI (32.9-89.2) for those with impaired LVEF at follow-up, 75.0% with 95% CI (46.3-89.8) for the unchanged LVEF group versus 95.8% with 95% CI (73.9-99.4) for the improved LVEF group.

At 5 years, these rates were 50.0% (95% CI (18.4-75.3)), 66.7% (95% CI (36.9-84.8)) and 81.2% (95% CI (56.9-92.6)) respectively.

In bivariate analysis (Figure 42), there was a statistically significant difference in the survival distributions of the impaired LVEF and improved LVEF groups (Log Rank < 10^{-3}).

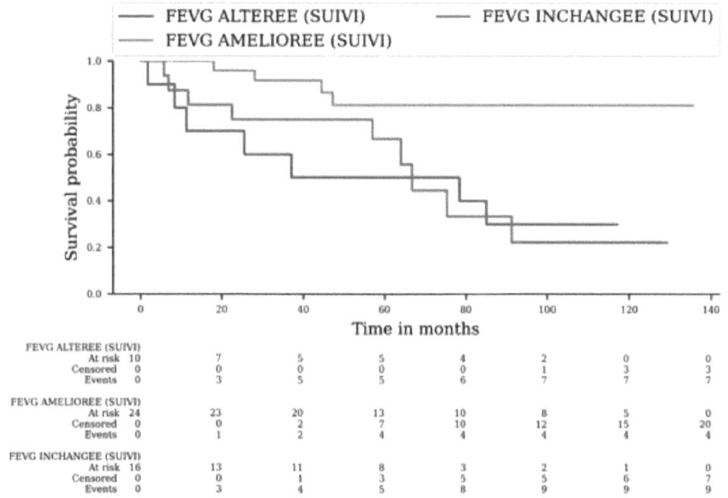

LVEF: Left ventricular ejection fraction

Figure 41 Analysis of survival as a function of late changes in ventricular ejection fraction

In multivariate Cox regression, LVEF deterioration during follow-up increased the risk of death five-fold (HR = 5.44 with a 95% CI of (1.92; 15.51); p=0.001).

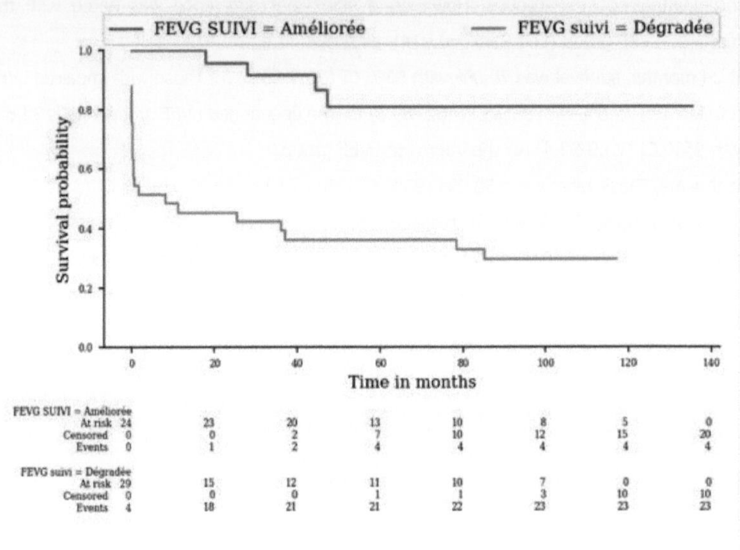

LVEF: Postoperative left ventricular ejection fraction

Figure 42 Binary analysis of survival as a function of late evolution of left ventricular ejection fraction (Improved Vs Degraded)

4.3. Analysis of the period free of major cardiovascular events

The median follow-up time was 96 months (extremes 19 months and 135 months) (Figure 43). Overall MACCE-free survival was 60.3% (95% CI (48.1; 74.0)) at 2 years and 43.8% (95% CI (31.9; 55.0)) at 5 years.

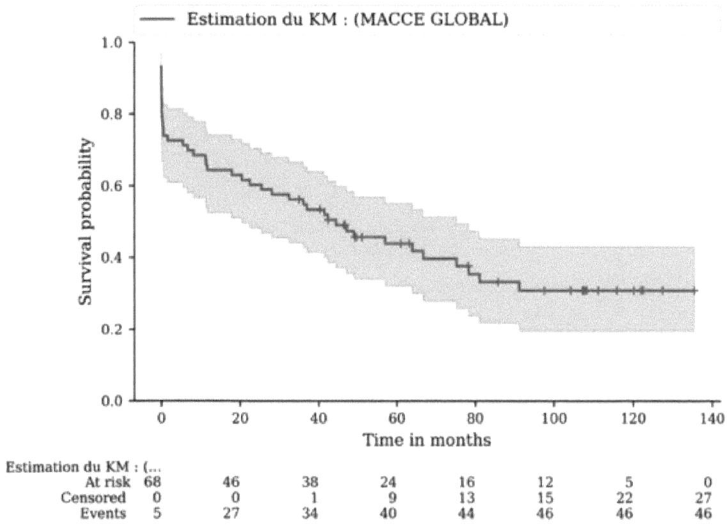

Estimation du KM : (...								
At risk	68	46	38	24	16	12	5	0
Censored	0	0	1	9	13	15	22	27
Events	5	27	34	40	44	46	46	46

Figure 43 Analysis of overall survival without major cardiovascular events

4.3.1. Comparative study of major cardiovascular event-free periods in patients with chronic kidney disease s

By comparing survival in renal failure patients with a GFR below 60 ml/min with those with a GFR greater than or equal to 60 ml/min, a significant difference was observed. Statistical comparison revealed a log Rank of 0.002, indicating a significant distinction between these two groups.

The MACCE-free survival curves for these respective categories can be seen in Figure 44, illustrating the disparities in survival rates according to renal function.

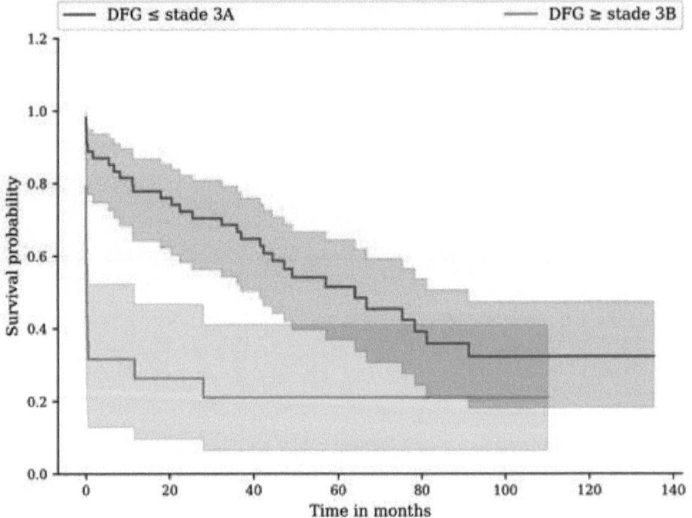

Figure 44 Analysis of major cardiovascular event-free survival in chronic renal failure

At 24 months: 26.3% (95% CI (9.6; 46.8)) versus 71.2% (95% CI (58.2; 82.2))

At 5 years and 60 months: 21.1% (95% CI (6.6; 41.0)) versus 51.5% (95% CI (36.9; 64.3))

4.3.2. Comparative study of major cardiovascular event-free periods in preoperative acute heart failure.

With regard to survival free of major cardiovascular events in patients with preoperative acute CHF, the analysis revealed no significant differences in survival curves between the different groups studied.

The Log-Rank value of 0.471 indicates that acute preoperative CI does not appear to influence survival free of major cardiovascular events in this patient population (Figure 45).

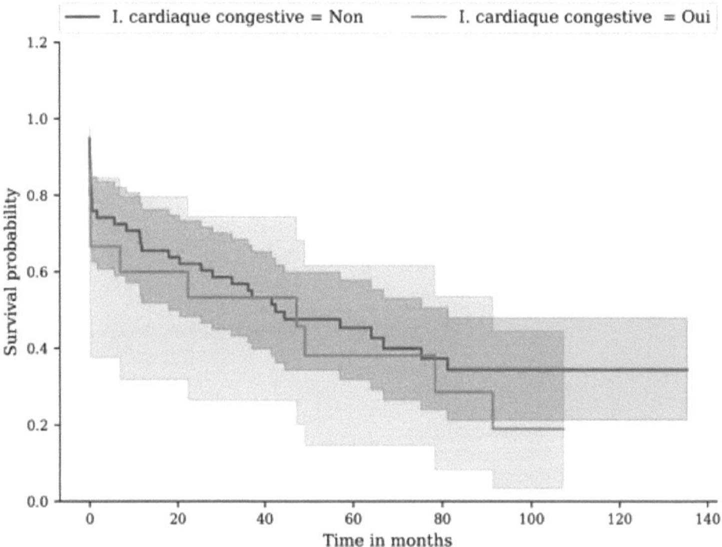

I. Cardiac: Heart failure

Figure 45 Analysis of major cardiovascular event-free survival in preoperative acute heart failure

4.3.3. Comparative study of major cardiovascular event-free periods in extreme emergency surgery.

In the case of extreme emergency surgery, analysis of survival free of major cardiovascular events revealed no significant differences in survival curves between the groups studied, as shown in figure 46. The Log-Rank value of 0.08 confirms the absence of any significant difference, indicating that performing surgery in an extreme emergency setting had no negative impact on 5-year major cardiovascular event-free survival.

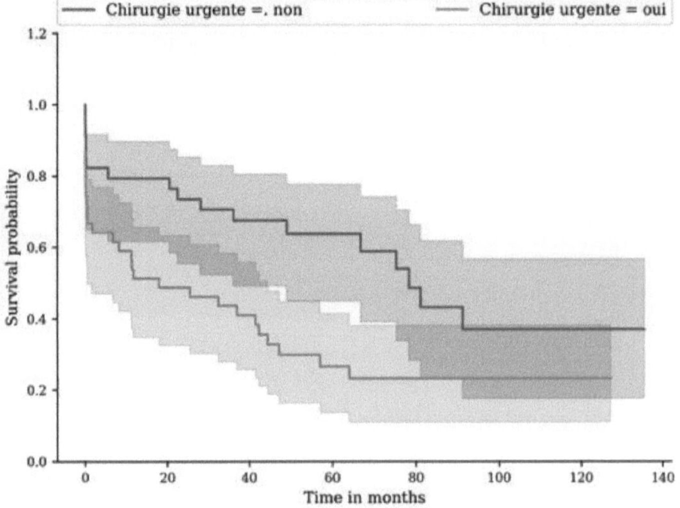

Figure 46 Analysis of survival free of major cardiovascular events in cases of extreme emergency coronary bypass surgery

4.3.4. Comparative study of Major Cardiovascular Event-Free Periods in postoperative infection.

Figure 47 shows that the occurrence of postoperative sepsis had an effect only on survival during the year following surgery, and that the two survival curves converged thereafter (log-Rank = 0.003).

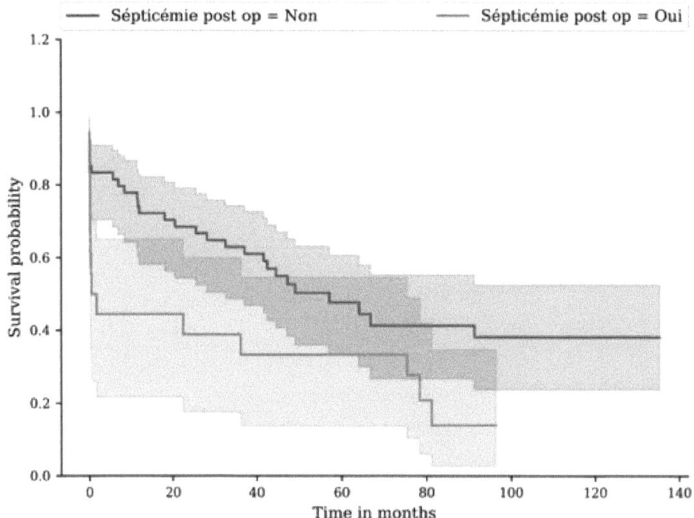

Figure 47 Analysis of major cardiovascular event-free survival in cases of postoperative sepsis

4.3.5. Comparative study of periods free of major cardiovascular events according to changes in left ventricular ejection fraction during follow-up :

Figure 48 shows a statistically significant difference during the first 5 years with better survival for the improved LVEF group (Log Rank <10).$^{-3}$

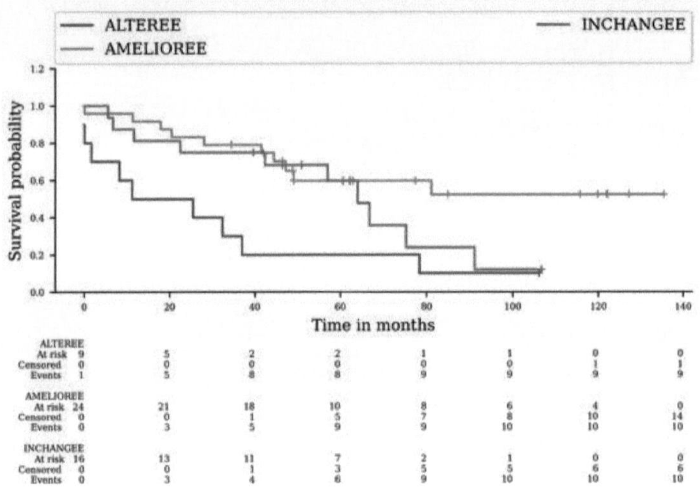

Figure 48 Analysis of major cardiovascular event-free survival as a function of changes in left ventricular ejection fraction

4.3.5.1. Multivariate analysis: Cox regression

In multivariate analysis, the independent factors that had an impact on MACCE-free survival curves are illustrated in Figure 49.

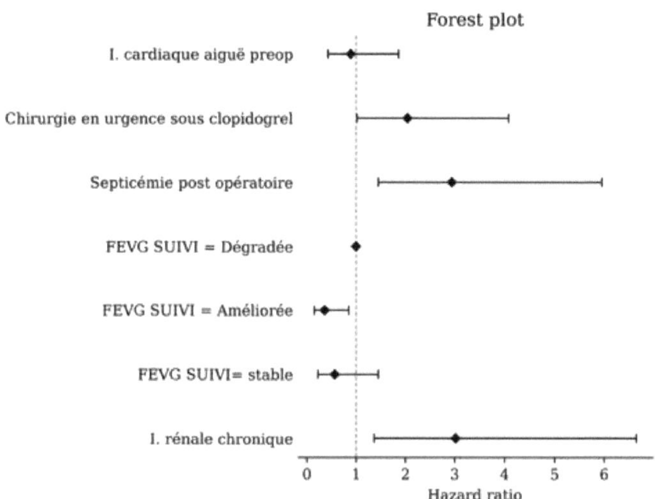

Figure 49 Factors predictive of late major cardiovascular events in multivariate analysis

Extreme emergency surgery: HR = 2.04 (95% CI (1.02; 4.08)); p = 0.04

Postoperative sepsis : HR = 2.94 (95% CI (1.45; 5.95)); p = 0.002

Chronic renal failure: HR = 3.02 (95% CI (1.37; 6.65)); p = 0.006

LVEF improvement at follow-up: HR = 0.36 (95% CI (0.152; 0.854)); p = 0.024

Discussions

The use of CABG in patients with coronary artery disease depends on factors such as clinical context, ventricular function, ischemic load and coronary anatomy. When coronary involvement is tritruncal, LV dysfunction is present, or there are large areas of ischemia, CABG is generally indicated[31].

Preoperative LV function is an important predictor of in-hospital mortality after CABG. Despite improvements in surgical techniques, myocardial protection and postoperative care, surgical risk in patients with reduced LV function remains high[32, 33].

In patients with decreased LVEF, CABG has shown better results than medical therapy alone, with improved symptoms and better survival [34, 35].

Advances in perioperative management, surgical techniques and myocardial protection methods have improved outcomes, encouraging practitioners to more readily opt for CABG in patients with reduced LVEF [36].

However, this could lead to perioperative SBDC and high postoperative mortality. Some patients may require inotropic or mechanical support for hours to days after surgery [37]. In addition, certain perioperative risk factors have been associated with reduced survival benefit and adverse events after CABG [38].

Identifying patients who could benefit most from surgical revascularization procedures remains a matter of debate.

The aim of our study was to investigate the immediate and medium-term mortality of coronary surgery in patients with ischemic heart disease with preoperative LV systolic dysfunction (preoperative LVEF≤ 40%).

According to the European Society of Cardiology (ESC) definition of CI [3]we set a threshold of 40% to identify patients with reduced LVEF. However, to broaden our sample and make our approach comparable with that of other national studies, we also included patients with an LVEF equal to 40%.

The main early postoperative cardiovascular events were early death (22%), postoperative SBDC (38%), postoperative acute coronary syndromes (16%) and stroke (1%). the predictive factors for early mortality were:

- ✓ Comorbidities: History of chronic renal failure or ACOMI
- ✓ Functional signs: The preoperative presence of NYHA III-IV exertional dyspnea.

- ✓ Coronary factors: the presence of tight TCG stenosis or multiple marginal lesions.
- ✓ Cardiovascular events: postoperative SBDC, postoperative myocardial infarction.
- ✓ Post-operative non-cardiovascular complications: acute renal failure, post-operative infection, need for mechanical ventilation for more than 10 hours.
- ✓ Postoperative echocardiographic factors: postoperative LVEF ≤ 33%.
- ✓ EuroSCORE II and STS risk scores had predictive thresholds for early mortality at 3.18% and 0.93%, respectively.

Among these factors, some were predictive of MACCE in particular:

- ✓ A history of chronic renal failure.
- ✓ The occurrence of a postoperative infectious complication.
- ✓ Post-operative LVEF ≤33%.
- ✓ Use of mechanical ventilation for more than 9 hours.

50 patients were followed up. The median follow-up was 95 months (8 years).

TTE at late follow-up showed that late left ventricular function improved in 24 patients (48%), was stable in 16 patients (32%), and was impaired in 10 patients (20%).

Factors predictive of mortality during follow-up were :

- ✓ Extreme emergency surgery with clopidogrel.
- ✓ Disturbances in anteroseptal segmental kinetics (preoperative).
- ✓ Mediastinitis.
- ✓ Poorly controlled diabetes at the time of cardiac surgery.
- ✓ Decrease in LVEF of at least 5%.

Factors predictive of MACCE during follow-up were:

- ✓ Chronic renal failure.
- ✓ Preoperative acute heart failure.
- ✓ Surgery in extreme emergency without stopping clopidogrel.
- ✓ The pre-existence of anteroseptal segmental kinetic disorders preoperatively.
- ✓ The occurrence of a postoperative infectious complication.

Conversely, improvement in LVEF ≥ 5% was associated with a better prognosis (OR= 0.2 (0.09; 0.8), p=0.049).

In multivariate analysis, the independent predictors of overall mortality were :

- ✓ The presence of kinetic disorders in the anterior or anteroseptal territory (OR=4.21; 95% CI (1; 15.77); p= 0.033).
- ✓ Extreme emergency surgery performed on clopidogrel (OR=1.1; 95% CI (1.45; 17.92); p= 0.011).
- ✓ Post-operative low cardiac output syndrome (OR=9.79; 95% CI (2.61; 36.75); p= 0.0007).

Survival analysis by Kaplan-Meier estimation showed that the overall survival of the cohort was 68.5% at 2 years and 57.9% at 5 years. In multivariate Cox regression, early postoperative LVEF impairment was found to be associated with a higher risk of mortality, with an HR of 3.62. AND deterioration in LVEF during follow-up was associated with a higher risk of mortality (HR =5.44).

LVEF improvement during follow-up was a protective factor associated with reduced MACCE and improved long-term survival in patients after surgical myocardial revascularization.

By taking LVEF trends into account, clinicians can better target therapeutic interventions and improve the overall management of patients after surgical myocardial revascularization. On the other hand, it is crucial to carefully monitor and treat post-operative complications such as infections and renal failure, as they increase the risk of morbidity and mortality. An improvement in LVEF during follow-up is also associated with a reduction in MACCE.

These findings can guide clinical decisions to improve patient survival after surgical myocardial revascularization. Careful monitoring of LVEF and consideration of risk factors should be key elements of patient management to optimize the outcome of this procedure.

Nevertheless, this study has certain limitations:

- ✓ The relatively small sample size and monocentric nature of the study limit the statistical power and generalizability of the results to a larger population.
- ✓ The retrospective nature of the study, based on medical records, could lead to selection and information bias, affecting the accuracy of the results.
- ✓ Delays in data collection could influence results due to missing or incomplete data.

- ✓ The absence of a comparison group makes it difficult to specifically assess the impact of left ventricular systolic dysfunction on postoperative morbidity and mortality.
- ✓ Changes in clinical practices and medical advances since the study period may limit the relevance of current results.

Despite these limitations, the results of this study could provide interesting insights into the predictors of morbidity and survival after surgical myocardial revascularization in cases of reduced LVEF. Further studies are needed to confirm and deepen our understanding of the clinical outcomes associated with this procedure.

1. Epidemiological analysis

Patients with coronary artery disease with severe LV dysfunction were considered inoperable, with an unfavorable prognosis and a two-year mortality of 69% [39-58]. However, thanks to technical advances in surgery, cardiac anesthesia and circulatory assistance, surgical revascularization is now being considered for these patients. According to the latest European recommendations on myocardial revascularization, beating-heart surgery is the option of choice in multitruncular patients with LVEF ≤ 35% [59]. Despite all this progress, mortality remains high in cases of LV dysfunction [8, 60, 61]. Thus, the debate persists as to the choice between surgical or endovascular revascularization, as well as the use of open-heart surgery in these fragile patients [60]. The threshold of LVEF≤40% was adopted to define reduced LVEF CI in this study thus approximating the definitions of the latest European chronic CI guidelines of 2021[3] while attempting to explore a niche of patients, with LVEF between 36 and 40%, not evoked by the 2018 European recommendations for myocardial revascularizations[2].

For LVEF ≤ 40%, the incidence rate at the main military training hospital in Tunis was 9.8 patients / 1000 PAC . Year. At the Habib Bourguiba Hospital in Sfax, the incidence rate was 36.7 patients/1000 PAC. Year [56] for the same LVEF threshold. In large international series, this incidence rate varied between 7.5 and 51 patients/1000 PAC. Year [40, 41, 43, 47-49, 62].

However, Table 20, comparing the main international studies, reveals heterogeneity in the LVEF threshold taken into consideration to define a CABG in LV dysfunction. This could be explained by the heterogeneity of the recommendations published at the time this work was carried out.

Considering only patients with LVEF ≤ 35% who had a CABG, the incidence rates were 8 and 4.1 patients/1000PAC.yr respectively at Sfax University Hospital [56] at HMPIT. These values are significantly lower than those reported in the international literature [2, 40, 41, 43, 47-49, 62] suggest a certain reluctance on the part of Tunisian heart teams to recommend surgical revascularization with bypass grafting and aortic clamping when LVEF falls below 35%.

In our two Tunisian studies, most patients underwent heart-stop bypass surgery. By adjusting the incidence rates of international studies according to the surgical strategy adopted, we observe that their figures are close to ours. This indicates a worldwide trend in favor of cardiac CB surgery for these patients, as illustrated in Table 20.

Table 20 Epidemiological profile of the main studies of coronary bypass surgery in the presence of left ventricular systolic dysfunction

Study	Country	Years of inclusion	Duration inclusion months	LV EF threshold (%)	Number of PAC	Number of PAC + LV dysfunction	Number of PAC + CEC heart stopped	LV dysfunction (%)	PAC + LV dysfunction incidence rate (/1000 PAC. YEAR)	Incidence rate of CABG under CEC + LV dysfunction (/1000 CABG. YEAR)
Kron et al. [39]	USA	1983-1988	72	<20	-	39	39	-	-	-
Elefteriades et al. [40]	USA	1981-1995	72	≤35	11830	744	744	6,2	10,4	10,4
Arom K.V. et al. [41]	USA	1998 - 1999	18	≤30	2303	177	132	7,6	51	38,2

Study	Country	Years of inclusion	Duration inclusion months	LV EF threshold (%)	Number of PAC	Number of PAC + LV dysfunction	Number of PAC + CEC heart stopped	LV dysfunction (%)	PAC + LV dysfunction incidence rate (/1000 PAC. YEAR)	Incidence rate of CABG under CEC + LV dysfunction (/1000 CABG. YEAR)
Shennib H. et al.[42]	Canada	1998 - 2001	46	≤35	-	77	46	-	-	-
Ascione R. et al. [43]	UK	1996-2002	76	≤30	5195	250	176	4,8	7,5	3,3
Hillis G.S. [44]	USA	1995-1999	5	<35	-	379	-	-	-	-
Darwazah A.K. et al. [45]	Jerusalem	2000-2004	48	≤35	-	150	84	-	-	-
Sharoni E. et al. [46]	Jerusalem	1999-2001	36	≤35	-	353	209	-	-	-
Wu et al [47]	Taiwan	1991-2002	144	<35	2842	365	365	12,8	10,7	10,7
Filsoufi F. et al. [48]	USA	1997-1999	36	≤30	2725	495	424	18,1	60,5	51,8
Youn T.N. et al.[49]	South Korea	2000-2005	60	<35	1473	153	53	10,4	20,7	3,5

Study	Country	Years of inclusion	Duration inclusion months	LV EF threshold (%)	Number of PAC	Number of PAC + LV dysfunction	Number of PAC + CEC heart stopped	LV dysfunction (%)	PAC + LV dysfunction incidence rate (/1000 PAC. YEAR)	Incidence rate of CABG under CEC + LV dysfunction (/1000 CABG. YEAR)
Attaran S.[50]	UK	1998-2009	120	≤30	-	943	528	-	-	-
Caputti G.M. et al. [51]	Brazil	2001-2005	60	≤20	-	217	112	-	-	-
Emmert M.Y. et al.[62]	Switzerland	2002-2008	84	<30	942	79	4	8,4	11,9	0,6
Keeling W.B. et al. [53]	USA	2008-2011	42	≤30	-	25667	20509	-	-	-
Ueki C. et al. [54]	Japan	2008-2012	60	≤30	-	2187	1134	-	-	-
Wang et al [55]	China	2013-2017	60	30-40	1152	112	44	9,7	19,4	7,6
Thesis MHIRI F. [56]	Tunisia	2010-2016	72	≤40	227	50	32	22,0	36,7	23,4
Tribak M. et al. [57]	Morocco	1995_2010	180	≤35	1434	171	137	11,9	7,9	6,3

Study	Country	Years of inclusion	Duration inclusion months	LV EF threshold (%)	Number of PAC	Number of PAC + LV dysfunction	Number of PAC + CEC heart stopped	LV dysfunction (%)	PAC + LV dysfunction incidence rate (/1000 PAC. YEAR)	Incidence rate of CABG under CEC + LV dysfunction (/1000 CABG. YEAR)
Our study	Tunisia	2012 - 2021	120	≤40	819	81	77	10	9,8	9,4

LVEF: Left ventricular ejection fraction, **CABG:** Coronary artery bypass graft, **LV:** Left ventricle

2. Clinical profile of coronary patients with left ventricular dysfunction

2.1. Age and gender

This study revealed a male predominance of 88%, with a female rate of 12%, in line with the majority of previously published studies (Table 21). On a national scale, the study by Mhiri F. [56] in Sfax found a female percentage of 24%, double that observed at HMPIT. The mean age of our patients was 60.5 ± 7.5 years, ranging from 40 to 80 years. These data are comparable with the various international and national studies reported in the literature and summarized in Table 21.

Age has been recognized as an independent risk factor affecting short- and medium-term mortality after CABG[63, 64]. Older patients may have more extensive coronary atherosclerosis, which may lead to increased mortality post CABG [65].

The lack of correlation between patient age and morbidity in our study could be explained by the relatively young age of our cohort.

Previously, age 65 was considered to be the point at which outcomes after CABG deteriorated, but thanks to technological advances and better patient selection, this threshold has been raised to age 80 [66-68].

Some studies have shown that female gender is an independent predictor of short-, medium- and long-term morbidity after CABG. [69-72].

Others have concluded that female gender was an independent risk factor for post CABG mortality, but was not an independent risk factor for postoperative morbidity [73]. Nevertheless, our results remain in line with some studies that have concluded that gender has no impact on outcomes after CABG. Indeed, some studies have found that female gender was not associated with excess mortality and had only a minimal impact on morbidity when patients were correctly matched[69, 74-76].

2.1. Risk factors cardiovascular

Our study, like others in the literature (Table 21), identified hypertension, diabetes and overweight as the main coronary risk factors. Compared with the study by Tribak et al. [57]our Tunisian sample showed a higher prevalence of hypertension (46.5% vs. 26.9%), but a lower prevalence of dyslipidemia (36% vs. 58.8%). Discrepancies in the prevalence of dyslipidemia may be due to varying definitions of this entity between studies.

2.1.1. Type 2 diabetes

There were no statistically significant associations between type 2 diabetes and post-PAC morbidity-mortality. However, Euroscore II considers diabetes on insulin as a predictor of 30-day post-PAC mortality [22].

2.1.2. Hypertension

No statistically significant correlation was found between hypertension and morbidity-mortality after CABG surgery with reduced LVEF, confirming the previous findings of Clough et al. [77]. Nevertheless, isolated hypertension has been associated with a 40% increase in the risk of postoperative morbidity in some studies [78]. Elevated pulse pressure has also been correlated with unfavorable outcomes [84]. Finally, it should be emphasized that hypertension has been identified as a risk factor for early mortality in hemodialysis patients undergoing CABG [79].

2.1.3. Overweight

58% of patients were overweight, with 18% obese. The median BMI was 26 kg/m^2 , ranging from 14 to 36 kg/m^2 . A further 3% of patients were underweight.

Overweight was not predictive of mortality or MACCE. However, it did correlate significantly with acute renal failure and postoperative infection.
These results are in partial agreement with the existing literature. It is generally accepted that obesity is a risk factor for postoperative complications and mortality in patients with LV dysfunction undergoing CABG [80-82]. Obesity, characterized by a BMI of 30 kg/m2 or more, has been associated with increased pulmonary morbidity following CABG [83] and severe obesity (BMI ≥ 40 kg/m2) has been identified as a risk factor for prolonged hospital stay [84].
However, the relationship between obesity and post-PAC outcomes remains unclear, with recent studies suggesting that increased BMI does not necessarily predict increased morbidity [85-88]. Some reports have indicated that only morbid obesity was an independent predictor of late mortality after CABG [89]. These controversial findings may be due to the inability to distinguish true excess body fat from developed muscle mass in patients with a slightly elevated BMI [90-92].
The impact of underweight on outcomes after CABG was also examined. Lean patients, with a BMI of less than 20 kg/m2, would have an increased risk of postoperative complications and mortality compared with normal-weight or overweight individuals [93, 94].

2.2. Coronary history s

We found a history of acute coronary events in 34% of patients, and 21% had undergone transluminal coronary angioplasty. This notion of a history of myocardial infarction has also been found in several studies of CABG with reduced LVEF. In a study by Youn T.N. et al. [49]51% of patients had a history of acute coronary events, including 14% with a history of TIA. Mhiri F. et al. [56] noted that 90% of their patients had had a myocardial infarction, and 24% had undergone percutaneous revascularization.
In a series of coronary artery bypass grafts in tritruncular diabetic patients, Nauffal et al. [95] observed that 5-year mortality was twice as high in tritruncular diabetics with a history of coronary angioplasty compared with the same population bypassed on native arteries. However, Nauffal et al. [95] found no increase in early mortality in this group. These results concur with those of Stevens et al.[96]who found no excess mortality at 30 days post CABG in patients who had undergone coronary angioplasty at least 15 days prior to surgery.

2.3. Other atheromatous vascular localizations

The prevalence of ACOMI in our study was 14%, which is in line with most published studies (3.6% to 24%). This is a higher proportion than that reported by Mhiri F. [56]which was six percent.

The prevalence of carotid atheroma was 21%, compared with a seven percent history of TIA and stroke not directly related to atheromatous carotid involvement.

On the one hand, our study identified ACOMI as a predictor of postoperative infection and early mortality in CABG in LV dysfunction. In agreement with some studies that have shown that ACOMI can affect the short- and long-term results of CABG surgery[97, 98].

On the other hand, carotid artery stenosis was not a predictor of mortality or MACCE, including stroke, possibly due to the limited sample size and low number of postoperative cerebrovascular events. It was, however, statistically significantly associated with postoperative infections.

In the literature, extracranial internal carotid artery stenosis is a risk factor for perioperative stroke in patients undergoing CABG surgery [99]. The risk of stroke ranges from 3% to 10% for a stenosis of 50% to 80%, and reaches 22% for a stenosis >80%. [100]. Preoperative screening by Doppler ultrasound of the carotid arteries is recommended for certain patients proposed for CABG, in particular those over 65 or with certain risk factors, such as tritruncal coronary disease, hypertension, CCOMI, smoking, previous stroke and diabetes. [101].

2.4. Chronic renal failure

The prevalence of CKD in our study was 23%, while Mhiri et al. [56] reported a higher prevalence of 62%. These results far exceed those observed in international studies of CABG in patients with reduced LVEF, where rates range from 4.5% to 13.2%. This difference could be explained by the high prevalence of arterial hypertension (AH) and diabetes in Tunisia, as well as less effective therapeutic management[102]. Indeed, it should be noted that only 51% of hypertensive patients reach their therapeutic objectives, according to data from the national NaTuRe HTN registry [102].

In addition, LV systolic dysfunction could give rise to a cardio-renal syndrome, which could contribute to the increased prevalence of CKD [103].

It should be noted that CKD influences the management of CABG and chronic heart failure by affecting drug prescription.[104]. An individualized approach is required, taking into account initial renal status and the severity of CKD.

CKD has been identified as a predictive factor for early mortality and late MACCE, consistent with the literature[103, 105]. However, we found no statistically significant correlation between mortality and CKD severity or transition to dialysis, despite the significant relationship between dialysis and postoperative infections. These results are in partial agreement with those of Minakata et al.[106]suggesting a correlation between risk of infection, early mortality and stage of CKD.

In the literature on CABG with reduced LVEF, CKD has been identified as a postoperative risk factor for cardiovascular complications, infections and mortality [105, 107-111].

Our results highlight the importance of multidisciplinary management to optimize the pre- and post-operative management of these patients.

2.5. Respiratory history

Fifteen percent of patients had chronic bronchitis, a prevalence very similar to those reported in the literature, which varies from 7.0% [57] à 12,8% [41].

COPD is common in patients undergoing CABG and can complicate perioperative management and prognosis. Despite the prevalence of COPD, our study did not demonstrate a statistical relationship between pulmonary history and postoperative morbidity and mortality. Our results are consistent with some studies [112, 113]. However, the literature recognizes COPD as a predictive factor of late post-PAC morbidity and mortality, particularly in severe forms undergoing systemic corticosteroid therapy or in patients over 75 years of age [114-116]. Indeed, this comorbidity could lead to various postoperative complications such as failure to wean patients from mechanical ventilation, sternal dehiscence, cardiac arrhythmias and prolongation of the length of stay in the intensive care unit[115].

Preventive treatment for moderate-risk COPD patients has been shown to be effective, improving postoperative outcomes and reducing complications and adverse events. Thus, a preoperative preparation protocol is recommended for patients scheduled to undergo CABG [117].

Table 21: Clinical characteristics of patients with left ventricular systolic dysfunction who have undergone coronary artery bypass grafting: Review of the literature

Study	Average age (years)	Women (%)	Smoking (%)	Type 2 diabetes (%)	HTA (%)	Dyslipidemia (%)	Overweight (%)	COPD (%)	CRI (%)	TIA/STROKE (%)	ACOMI (%)	HISTORY OF MI (%)	ATCDATL (%)
Arom K.V. et al. [41]	66± 11.6	15,3	18,8	33,8	53,4	-	7,5	12,8	-	-	12,0	-	-
Shennib H. et al.[42]	64.5 ± 9.9	5,2	29,0	41,9	41,9	54,8	-	3,2	9,7	6,5	6,5	74,2	-
Ascione R. et al. [43]	65,0	4,0	75,0	23,0	53,0	74,0	-	9,0	-	15,0	17,0	79,0	-
Hillis G.S. [44]	69	24,0	21	40	65	-	-	-	52	-	-	69	16
Darwaza	58.7 ± 9.4	16,7	52,4	52,4	45,2	31,0	-	9,5	9,5	4,8	3,6	50,0	-

Study	Average age (years)	Women (%)	Smoking (%)	Type 2 diabetes (%)	HTA (%)	Dyslipidemia (%)	Overweight (%)	COPD (%)	CRI (%)	TIA/STROKE (%)	ACOMI (%)	HISTORY OF MI (%)	ATCDATL (%)
h A.K. et al. [45]													
Sharoni E. et al. [46]	63.0 ± 10.6	10,2	35,0	38,0	68,0	-	-	23,0	12,0	-	-	77,0	4
Wu et al [47]	60.5 ± 7.5	7,9	47,4	38,9	62,5	27,7	-	7,1	13,2	8,5	10,7	57,5	17,5
Filsoufi F. et al. [48]	65.0 ± 11.0	23,6	-	46,0	77,0	-	20,0	10,0	8,0	8,0	19,0	78,0	14
Youn T.N. et al.[49]	62.0 ± 9.2	9,8	37,7	49,1	49,1	41,5	3,8	5,7	13,2	7,5	11,3	50,9	13,2
Attaran S.[50]	66,1	14,8	19,5	32,5	61,8	92,4	-	42,4	12,6	11,1	20,2	17,0	-
Caputti	67.0 ± 2.0	10,6	25,9	33,9	52,7	42,8	7,1*	11,6	8,9	7,1	12,5	35,7	-

Study	Average age (years)	Women (%)	Smoking (%)	Type 2 diabetes (%)	HTA (%)	Dyslipidemia (%)	Overweight (%)	COPD (%)	CRI (%)	TIA/STROKE (%)	ACOMI (%)	HISTORY OF MI (%)	ATCDATL (%)
G.M. et al. [51]													
Emmert M.Y. et al.[62]	63.0 ± 9.0	23	59	48	24	-	-	3,0	-	-	12,0	39,0	-
Keeling W.B. et al. [53]	64,0	16,1	-	52,3	84,1	-	-	33,1	-	16,0	19,1	66,5	-
Ueki C. et al. [54, 118]	65.7 ± 10.2	7,1	65,4	64,5	73,6	59	-	10,6	-	13,2	18,7	61,1	24,6
Wang et al [55]	61	11,6	47,7	15,9	63,6	72,7	56,8	11,3	4,5	63,6	-	65,9	11,3
Thesis MHI	63,5	24,0	70,0	58,0	58,0	30,0	30,0	-	62,0	6,0	6,0	90,0	24,0

Study	Average age (years)	Women (%)	Smoking (%)	Type 2 diabetes (%)	HTA (%)	Dyslipidemia (%)	Overweight (%)	COPD (%)	CRI (%)	TIA/STROKE (%)	ACOMI (%)	HISTORY OF MI (%)	ATCDATL (%)
RI F. [56]													
Tribak M. et al. [57]	57,5 ± 7,6	7,0	58,8	48,5	26,9	58,8	7	1,7	-	2,9	24,5	85,3	12,2
Our study	**60,5 ±7,5**	**12**	**69,0**	**54,7**	**46,5**	**36,0**	**58,8**	**15,0**	**23,2**	**6,8**	**13,6**	**34,2**	**20,5**

CCOA: Chronic obliterative arteriopathy of the lower limbs, **TIA:** Transient ischemic attack, **Past** history, **TAA:** Transluminal angioplasty**, Stroke:** Cerebrovascular accident, **COPD:** Chronic obstructive pulmonary disease, **HTA:** Hypertension, **MI:** Myocardial infarction**, CKD:** Chronic renal failure.

2.1. Clinical presentation

2.1.1. Circumstances of discovery

In this study, the prevalence was 52% for NSTEMI, 18% for STEMI and four percent for chronic coronary syndrome. Of the 27% of patients with clinical signs of preoperative acute congestive heart failure, 90% were admitted for myocardial infarction. These rates were similar to those at Sfax University Hospital [56] which were 56% for NSTEMI, 16% for STEMI and 8% for chronic coronary syndrome.

In two recent Canadian studies of myocardial revascularization in patients with reduced LVEF [119, 120]the clinical presentation of patients proposed for CABG was dominated by myocardial infarction (39%) in the province of Alberta, whereas in Toronto, chronic coronary syndromes were more frequent (37.2%). These variations suggest an influence of healthcare system and geographic region on the circumstances of discovery of severe ischemic heart disease with reduced LVEF.

In terms of morbidity and mortality, post-SCA CABG in extreme emergency was a predictor of mortality and late MACCE in our study. On the other hand, the presence of preoperative acute CHF was predictive of increased early mortality and later MACCE.

Our results were divergent compared to some data in the literature which concluded that ACS was associated with early postoperative excess mortality only, with long-term outcomes comparable to those of stable angina [121].

Indeed, emergency CABG with bypass grafting and aortic clamping induces ischemia followed by myocardial reperfusion on already ischemic and sometimes siderated myocardium, amplifying the territory of myocardial lesions. This is proportional to the duration of bypass surgery and aortic clamping. This situation complicates the exit from bypass surgery, often necessitating the use of catecholamines. However, catecholamines, while increasing myocardial afterload and metabolic requirements, can cause splanchnic vasoconstriction and acidosis. This acidosis reduces the heart's sensitivity to catecholamines, creating a deleterious vicious circle. While the use of circulatory assistance may be a solution to counteract this phenomenon, it also introduces its own set of potential complications.

According to O'Boyle et al, an increased incidence of major cardiac events and higher in-hospital mortality is observed in patients with preoperative Troponin I_C >0.15ng/ml [122]. The three-month threshold between ACS and CABG is one of the parameters used to estimate early mortality using the Euroscore II, underlining that bypass surgery performed within three months of a myocardial infarction carries a higher risk than earlier infarctions. [22]. In a recent study, it was found that patients operated on within the first 48 hours of a myocardial infarction had a similar mortality rate to those operated on between days three and seven, suggesting that it may be feasible to shorten the time between myocardial infarction and CABG for some patients [123]. According to a meta-analysis by Lang et al.[124] in 2022, it is recommended, if possible, to delay CABG for at least 24 hours after myocardial infarction. However, the timing of this bypass does not appear to influence mortality in patients with NSTEMI. Furthermore, no statistical difference was observed in perioperative myocardial infarction or stroke between early and late procedures[124].

2.1.2. Examination physical

The presence of NHYA 3 exertional dyspnea was a risk factor for early postoperative mortality. These results are consistent with those of Larusso et al. who showed that advanced NYHA III or IV preoperative dyspnea were independent risk factors for early postoperative mortality[125].

3. Further tests

3.1. Complementary non-invasive tests

3.1.1. Data from electrocardiogram

Five percent had atrial fibrillation, which is consistent with the prevalences observed in other series in the literature, generally varying between 5 and 12% [51, 56, 57]. With regard to complete left bundle branch block (CLBBB), seven percent of patients had this conductive disorder, which was similar to the 6% rate reported by Mhiri et al.[56].

3.1.2. Preoperative biology data

3.1.2.1. Preoperative anemia

In this study, 16% of patients had preoperative anemia. This condition, particularly during cardiac surgery under CEC, may increase the risk of complications due to a reduction in the blood's ability to carry oxygen[126]. In addition, CEC itself can cause haemodilution, which can lead to anaemia even in patients without pre-existing anaemia.

Complications associated with anemia during and after coronary surgery with CEC include increased risk of infection, impaired immune function, impaired cardiac function, as well as prolonged hospital stay and increased mortality [127]. One of the main consequences of anemia is the need for transfusion. If transfusion is intrinsically harmful, it is all the more so in a context of intense inflammation induced by bypass surgery. Numerous studies have shown that transfusion of more than two bags is predictive of morbidity and mortality.[128, 129]. It is therefore important to check for the presence of anemia preoperatively, taking into account the urgency of the situation. The aim of this approach is not only to treat the anemia to prevent its adverse effects, but also to identify the cause, which could be a condition favoring bleeding in the context of CEC associated with heparin.[130]

During the pre-operative phase, it is also important to optimize the patient's hematological status, including the correction of deficiencies in iron, vitamin B12 and red blood cell production factors. During surgery, autotransfusion techniques can be used to manage anemia [131].

3.1.2.2. Preoperative glycated hemoglobin

Ninety-five percent of diabetic patients had poorly controlled diabetes prior to surgery, with a mean HbA1c of 8.9±2.2%. This parameter had good sensitivity and specificity for predicting late mortality, and an HbA1c > 9% had an OR = 30. These results concur with those of Agarwal GR et al. [132] who found that HbA1c > 8% was predictive of mortality with an OR = 3.25, as well as other studies which have demonstrated a fourfold increase in mortality risk for HbA1c > 8% [133]. These data confirm the crucial need for optimal glycemic control prior to surgery. High HbA1c is associated with an increased risk of postoperative complications and death. Indeed, poorly controlled diabetes is predictive of mediastinitis, a severe infection characterized by high morbidity and mortality.

The choice of heart graft should also take this parameter into account. If the patient has poorly controlled diabetes, it is recommended to avoid the use of a double breast graft, as this could increase the risk of mediastinitis. However, it is important to note that poorly controlled diabetes is not an absolute contraindication, but it does carry documented and significant risks [134]. For stable patients, any intervention should be deferred until diabetes is under control, which is essential to improve results and minimize risks.

Furthermore, patients with type 2 diabetes on insulin had a higher mortality rate and a higher post-CAP MACCE rate than patients treated with oral antidiabetics [135].

In our study, preoperative HbA1c was not identified as a significant predictor of early morbidity or mortality. These observations are consistent with the findings of some studies suggesting that immediate outcomes after CABG in diabetic patients are not necessarily influenced by the level of preoperative glycemic control or therapeutic modality, but rather by rigorous perioperative glycemic monitoring [136]. In addition, optimal management of diabetes mellitus, associated cardiovascular comorbidities and smoking cessation are key factors in maximizing long-term survival in this population. [137, 138].

3.2. Echocardiographic data

3.2.1. Preoperative left ventricular systolic ejection fraction

Sixty-four percent of patients had LVEF between 36% and 40%, while 36% had LVEF ≤ 35%. These results were close to those of Mhiri et al. [56] who observed proportions of 78% and 22% respectively.

The mean LVEF observed in our study was 37 ± 3%, which is close to the means reported by other studies adopting the same research methodology (LVEF ≤ 40%). For example, Wang et al. [55] found a mean LVEF of 34.9 ± 4.5%, while Mhiri et al. [56] reported a value of 34.9%.

It is well established that preoperative LVEF is an important predictor of early and late mortality after CABG. Despite advances in therapeutics and surgical techniques, the management of patients with reduced LVEF still remains a challenge [36, 44, 139].

Current risk scores (Euroscore II, STS score) identify LVEF as a powerful predictor of intraoperative and 30-day mortality [22, 140].

According to current research, a reduced preoperative LVEF is a major indicator of post CABG complications. Indeed, the performance of this procedure under aortic clamping is associated with a significant morbi-mortality, as this technique imposes myocardial ischemia. When the clamp is lifted, myocardial sideration sets in, an inescapable consequence of the prior ischemia. The extent of this sideration is directly correlated with the duration of clamping, and modulated by the quality of myocardial protection provided during the surgical procedure.

In the case of a previously collapsed LVEF, the clinical repercussions may become evident as early as the first hours postoperatively. This can result in left ventricular failure, sometimes progressing to postoperative low cardiac output syndrome, or even fatal refractory cardiogenic shock.

The development of any of these complications will undoubtedly prolong the patient's stay in the intensive care unit and the need for mechanical ventilation, further exposing the patient to nosocomial complications, among which infectious pneumonitis stands out. Moreover, in this context of cardiac fragility, infections may be particularly serious. Indeed, the oxidative stress induced by sepsis, combined with increased metabolic requirements and impaired oxygen extraction, would put the heart to the test. An already failing myocardium would have difficulty meeting these increased demands, which could worsen the clinical picture [141-143].

The impact of the numerical value of preoperative LVEF on postoperative morbidity and mortality could not be established in this work. This limitation may stem from the study design, which included only patients with reduced LVEF, the predominance of patients with 40% LVEF, and the small sample size.

In patients with LVEF ≤ 35%, CABG has proved superior to medical treatment alone. It improved quality of life and increased long-term survival, as demonstrated by the landmark Coronary Artery Surgery Study (CASS) [144] and more recently the Surgical Treatment for Ischemic Heart Failure (STICH) trial [35, 61].

3.2.2. Study of myocardial viability

The study of hibernating myocardium is fundamental to assess the reversibility of LV dysfunction after myocardial reperfusion. Several imaging methods, such as dobutamine echocardiography, myocardial scintigraphy and cardiac MRI, have been proposed [145]. These examinations also facilitate the selection of patients eligible for myocardial revascularization in cases of severe ventricular dysfunction, and could potentially simplify the surgical procedure by reducing the number of coronary axes targeted for bypass surgery [57, 146].

In this study, 52% of patients showed severe myocardial akinesia or hypokinesia on resting echocardiography. However, only one in four patients had this assessment. These figures are close to the results of the study by Mhiri et al. and are below what has been reported by Moroccan and other international studies [57, 147].

The impact of the presence of myocardial viability on the revascularization and survival of patients with ischemic cardiomyopathy is the subject of much debate. While some studies have demonstrated its importance in predicting functional improvement after revascularization, others, such as the STICH trial, have questioned its prognostic impact [148].

The STICH trial, involving 1221 patients at 99 sites in 22 countries over a 10-year period, compared coronary artery bypass grafting with medical therapy in patients with ischemic heart disease with LVEF≤35% [8, 61]. It found no significant survival benefit in patients with myocardial viability undergoing revascularization compared with those receiving optimal medical therapy alone [148]. However, this trial has its limitations, notably the pooling of results from different imaging techniques despite their differences in specificity[148]. Despite the results of the STICH trial, other studies have confirmed the benefits of revascularization of viable myocardial territories identified by imaging techniques such as dobutamine stress echocardiography [149-155].

In this study, cardiac viability tests were essential for surgical decisions:

1. Determining the need for bypass surgery: Viability in certain areas supported the decision to bypass.
2. Optimizing the surgical approach: In other situations, the lack of viability has influenced the decision to limit the number of grafts, enabling a more targeted, shorter and potentially less risky procedure.
3. Evaluating infarction and revascularization: certain tests helped to identify the infarct's condition. Indeed, cardiac MRI revealed microvascular obstruction, hence the failure to place a bridge downstream of the chronic occlusion of the coronary artery serving this non-viable territory.

In conclusion, cardiac viability testing has enabled an accurate and tailored assessment of myocardial status in patients with various coronary diseases. This information has been instrumental in guiding and optimizing surgical decisions, enabling more targeted and potentially more effective interventions [57, 147].

3.3. Additional invasive tests

3.3.1. Coronary angiography data

Eighty-two patients had tritruncular lesions and 19% a severe lesion (>50%) of the TCG, while mono or bi-truncular lesions accounted for only 8% of cases. Tritroncular status or a TCG lesion were predictive of early postoperative mortality, in agreement with data in the literature [156].

Looking at Table 22, we see that the majority of patients with LV dysfunction referred for cardiac surgery were tritruncal. These results are broadly consistent with other international studies.

Table 22 Analysis of the distribution of patients' coronary status according to the literature.

Study	Truncular status MONO	BI	TRI	TCG+
Hillis G.S. et al. **[44]**	_	_	81	32
Darwazah A.K. et al. **[45]**	6	18	76	_
Sharoni E. et al. **[46]**	55	20	74	_
Wu et al **[47]**	4	16	80	17
Filsoufi F. et al. **[48]**	4	18	78	
Youn T.N. et al.**[49]**	_	_	87	30
Attaran S.**[50]**	_	_	90	_
Ueki C. et al. **[118]**	_	_	84	36
Wang et al **[55]**	1	7	92	25
Mickleborough L. et al. **[157]**	2	18	80	11
Thesis MHIRI F. **[56]**	6	28	66	44
Tribak M. et al. **[57]**	4	25	70	18
Our study	**1**	**17**	**82**	**19**

TCG+: Involvement of the left common coronary trunk

Although our study showed no significant direct correlation between overall mortality and coronary calcification, this factor was predictive of postoperative LVEF deterioration. An independent predictor of mortality.

These results are in agreement with previous work, such as that by Ertelt et al. [158]where the presence of severe coronary calcifications was an independent predictor of adverse ischemic outcomes, including MACCE and mortality or myocardial infarction.

Our results could be explained by the fact that calcification reduces vascular elasticity, thus affecting coronary perfusion and vasomotor functions. Despite effective bypass surgery, distal endothelial dysfunction, a poor distal bed and calcified emboli may increase the rate of ischemia. In addition, severely calcified vessels may make vascular anastomoses more complex, lengthen procedure time and reduce graft quality[158, 159]. Calcification may also limit complete revascularization, which is generally associated with better long-term results. Finally, severe calcification may indicate aggressive systemic atherosclerosis, associated with a poor prognosis [158, 159].

It should be noted that the presence of significant calcifications or iterative stent restenosis can pose technical challenges during percutaneous coronary dilation procedures, which may reduce their effectiveness or increase risks. In these situations, cardiac surgery may be considered a more appropriate alternative to ensure adequate revascularization[2].

In conclusion, it is essential to take into account the patient's individual profile, available resources, and potential risks and benefits when choosing the optimal treatment. A shared decision between the patient and the medical team, based on a thorough assessment of the clinical situation and available options, is crucial in determining the best therapeutic approach in each specific case.

3.4. Antiplatelet therapy

Sixty percent of patients admitted for ACS received clopidogrel as pre-treatment prior to coronary angiography, with this treatment usually discontinued five days before the procedure. In fact, in patients scheduled for CABG less than 5 days after the last clopidogrel treatment, a significantly higher incidence of reinterventions, major bleeding and bleeding-related complications was observed. [160].

Coronary surgery on clopidogrel should therefore be reserved for extreme emergencies. An individualized approach based on the clinical context of each patient may be necessary to guide therapeutic decision-making.

3.4.1. Treatment of chronic heart failure

This study reveals insufficient treatment of CHF in patients prior to cardiac surgery. Only 92% of patients were taking beta-blockers and ACE inhibitors, and less than 80% were receiving a beta-blocker specifically validated for CHF. Moreover, only 15% of patients were prescribed anti-aldosterone. In addition, 27% showed signs of cardiac congestion requiring a loop diuretic at the time of surgery.

According to the latest ESC recommendations [3]this treatment was suboptimal. However, it is important to note that our study took place over a 10-year period, from 2012 to 2021, during which recommendations have followed one another, leading to a rapid evolution in protocols and initiation times for IC treatment. These factors may partly explain the observed under-treatment. It is also important to mention that 70% of patients underwent CABG as a result of acute coronary syndrome, leaving little time for treatment optimization prior to surgery.

In order to improve the management of CHF prior to surgery, it is essential to adhere to the current ESC recommendations on drug therapy for chronic CHF. The timing of surgery must also be considered, requiring close collaboration between cardiologists and cardiac surgeons to adapt preoperative treatment to the time available. A thorough preoperative examination, including assessment of LV function and congestion, is essential to determine the best treatment strategies. Future studies could also assess the impact of preoperative IC treatment optimization protocols on postoperative outcomes.

3.4.2. Preoperative hemodynamic support

In this study, seven percent of patients received preoperative Levosimendan prophylaxis, and one patient was treated with dobutamine before being switched to Levosimendan due to a preoperative low cardiac output condition.

Levosimendan is a calcium sensitizer that activates the adenosine triphosphate (ATP)-dependent potassium channel and possesses positive inotropic, vasodilatory and cardioprotective properties[161, 162]. It increases cardiomyocyte sensitivity to calcium and may also prolong its pharmacodynamic effects through inhibition of phosphodiesterase III [163].

In addition to its initial indication for acute decompensated IC, it is also used for its beneficial effect on renal function [164, 165].

A meta-analysis by Harrison et al. indicated that Levosimendan use is associated with a reduction in mortality, with a more pronounced benefit in patients with reduced LVEF[166].

Recently, three multicenter randomized placebo-controlled clinical trials (LICORN[167]CHEETAH[168] and LEVO-CTS[169]) have been published. The LICORN[167]which evaluated the efficacy of Levosimendan in reducing the incidence of postoperative SBDC in 336 patients with LVEF ≤ 40% undergoing CABG, failed to reach statistical significance for the composite primary endpoint. Nevertheless, among the secondary endpoints, the duration of postoperative catecholamine therapy was shorter in the Levosimendan group[167].

The CHEETAH[168]and LEVO-CTS[169] showed no significant difference in 30-day mortality between the Levosimendan and placebo groups in patients with postoperative SBDC. However, patients treated with Levosimendan had fewer postoperative low cardiac output events and required less inotropic support than the placebo group.

Based on these data, an expert opinion in 2018[170] concluded that Levosimendan is a safe and effective agent for the treatment of patients undergoing cardiac surgery requiring inotropic support. However, mortality benefits were statistically significant only in certain subgroups, such as patients undergoing isolated CABG and those with reduced LVEF. The same finding was established in 2022 by Caruba et al.[171].

Despite some positive results, the effect of Levosimendan is not as great as assumed in earlier studies. Consequently, this molecule cannot be recommended for routine use at the present time, especially in view of its high cost. [170].

A recent study evaluated the impact of the timing of Levosimendan administration in high-risk SBDC patients undergoing cardiac surgery. Preoperative administration of Levosimendan significantly reduced in-hospital mortality, as well as the duration of mechanical ventilation and the need for renal replacement therapy. This suggests that "reconditioning" with Levosimendan could be beneficial in these high-risk patients. However, further randomized clinical trials are needed to confirm these promising results[172].

3.5. Preoperative prediction of early mortality by Euroscore II and STS score

Since the 2011 revision, the Euroscore II has been widely used in Europe to estimate the risk of mortality within 30 days after cardiac surgery. [20-22]. In our study, the mean risk of mortality predicted by Euroscore II was 2.81 ± 2.1%, with a median of 2%, whereas actual 30-day mortality was 20%.

In the Moroccan study by Tribak et al.[57]this mean was 2.3 ± 1.9 (0.7-13). Another study by Mhiri et al. [56] at the CHU Habib Bourguiba in Sfax showed an average theoretical risk of 2.8%, with an actual intraoperative mortality of 4%.

In 2018, Bouabdallaoui et al. [173] attempted to recalculate operative risk prediction scores, focusing in particular on the Euroscore II and STS score, for the 814 patients in the STICH trial between 2002 and 2007. The median Euroscore II in the two groups was 2.4% and 2.9% respectively, with actual 30-day mortality of 4.8% and 3.5%.

For the STS score, in our study, the predicted mean 30-day mortality was 1.3 ± 1.07%, with extremes of 0.42% and 6.69%, and a median of 0.88%. This risk was underestimated compared with Euroscore II. Bouabdallaoui et al. [173] found that the STS score also underestimated predicted mortality compared with Euroscore II.

It appears that predictive 30-day mortality scores, such as the Euroscore II and STS score, give less accurate results for specific high-risk subpopulations, such as those with impaired LVEF. This could be explained by the fact that these models were not designed to accurately assess the risk of surgical mortality in specific subgroups where certain risk factors, not included in these scores, are predominant. However, this finding is subject to debate among researchers to this day [173].

In the context of this research, both scores - Euroscore II and STS - demonstrated a significant statistical correlation with mortality and major short-term cardiovascular events. However, in order to establish a precise and relevant mortality prediction threshold for the Tunisian population, further investigation through registry studies is imperative.

3.6. Surgical revascularization

3.6.1. Operating time

In our study, the mean time to surgical myocardial revascularization was 62 ± 52 days after coronary angiography, a range comparable to that observed in the study by Mhiri et al. [56]where it was 57.9 ± 61.9 days.

However, patients with TCG stenosis were operated on rapidly even in the absence of extreme emergency situations.

Some authors have studied the evolution of patients in the days leading up to surgery, in an attempt to identify poor prognostic factors and indications for urgent surgery.

Maziak et al. [174] suggested that surgery within 10 days of diagnosis for patients with significant TCG stenosis did not decrease the rate of mortality or major cardiac complications, and also suggested that stable patients can wait for surgery without increased risk of complications. In contrast, Da Rocha et al. [175] identified acute coronary syndrome as a predictive factor for mortality and cardiovascular events, requiring urgent intervention.

3.6.1. Myocardial protection :

The operative strategy was identical for all patients in our study: surgery under extracorporeal circulation, aortic clamping and myocardial protection by cold blood cardioplegia administered anterogradely, in moderate hypothermia followed by terminal reperfusion with warm blood. This is a classic approach, widely used worldwide and mastered by the team.

Since the first description of reversible chemical cardiac arrest in 1955 by Melrose [176]and the first myocardial protection in 1956 by Lillehe [177]myocardial protection has been at the heart of innovation in cardiac surgery. Obtaining a bloodless, immobile surgical field implies the use of a highly non-physiological procedure represented by bypass grafting and aortic clamping. This procedure is associated with a large number of undesirable effects, the most critical of which is cardiac ischemia-reperfusion, responsible for myocardial sideration or necrosis.

These phenomena are exacerbated in hearts prone to ischemia due to coronary lesions, and the consequences are all the more serious in cases of preoperative ventricular dysfunction.

After 70 years of innovation, several options are available to the surgical team to ensure myocardial protection under aortic clamping. These include cardioplegia solutions, administration procedures and pharmacological means.

Cardioplegia using pure crystalloid solutions (with or without metabolites and buffers) is still used in cardiac surgery. Although these solutions were the first to be adopted, they have been criticized for their poor buffering and oxygen-carrying capacity in the absence of blood.

Cardioplegia with blood allows reoxygenation of the heart during cardioplegic arrest, limits hemodilution, offers superior buffering capacity and optimized osmolarity, ensures physiological ph, contains antioxidant and anti-free radical elements and offers exemplary ease of use, given that these are natural characteristics of blood. Despite this number of undeniable theoretical advantages, studies have not shown unanimous superiority [178-181]and several meta-analyses have concluded that the two solutions are equivalent in terms of mortality and postoperative MI, even if enzymatic or anatomopathological differences have been demonstrated[182, 183]

A large number of cardioplegia solutions exist, including microplegia[184]or the Del Nido solution[185]These offer multiple advantages, but their clinical impact still varies from study to study (mostly small-scale studies), which does not allow for a high level of proof. Similarly, the temperature of administration of the cardioplegia solution - cold, warm or hot - has also been a subject of debate, without conclusive results[186]. It is important to point out, however, that the most physiological means (blood solutions, at a temperature as close to normal as possible) should be preferred for the most at-risk subgroups, such as patients with LV dysfunction.

The route of cardioplegia administration is also important to consider, particularly in the presence of coronary lesions of the left common trunk or tritruncal lesions.

These complex, diffuse and sometimes occlusive coronary lesions lead to non-uniform distribution of the solution in the coronary bed and myocardium, at least in theory, via the classic anterograde (aortic root) route. This can be compensated for by the retrograde route through the coronary sinus. However, there are a number of disadvantages:

- The need for specific (more onerous) cannulas to be implanted through the right atrium under TEE guidance, or the need to open the right atrium.
- The risk of coronary sinus lesions, which can be complex to repair.
- Inconsistent perfusion of the anterior wall of the VD, due to insufficient drainage by the coronary sinus and the minimal veins (of Thebesius) draining directly into the right cavities, and the great anatomical variability of the venous system [187]

Studies have shown that the retrograde route is effective and risk-free, but its superiority to the anterograde route remains to be proven.[188].

The combination of anterograde and retrograde routes represents a compromise that compensates for the shortcomings of the different methods. Administration via venous grafts can also be combined with these two routes. This multimodal approach has shown interesting results in several studies, especially in cases of severe coronary lesions or LV dysfunction[189-191]. However, it is necessary to consider the constraints and complexity of deploying such techniques.

There are also a large number of pharmacological means of myocardial protection, such as adenosine, sodium-hydrogen exchanger inhibitors, acadesin, the glucose-insulin-potassium combination or cyclosporine, whose efficacy has been inconsistent.

A review of the literature shows that myocardial protection methods are numerous, with specific advantages and disadvantages, and can be combined in highly variable ways. It is therefore more appropriate to speak of myocardial protection strategies, to be adopted and mastered by surgical teams and modulated according to patient characteristics, while ensuring that the greatest importance is attached to aortic clamping and bypass times, the main links in the chain of adverse effects.

Beating-heart surgical myocardial revascularization is also a solution to the harmful consequences of aortic clamping, but also to emboligenic aortic manipulation, organ failure and bleeding complications. It can also be integrated into minimally invasive or robotic solutions that are highly demanding in logistical and financial terms. Although expertise in this technique has evolved over the years, leading to improved results [192]The results are not conclusive. Reservations have been expressed regarding the rate of incomplete revascularization, postoperative MI and graft patency[193, 194]. Clinical interest in LV dysfunction is also controversial, in line with the reservations already cited [195-199]. This explains the ESC recommendations that this practice should be reserved for high-volume centers [2]This also applies to minimally invasive and robotic techniques. These are mainly hybrid techniques combining surgical revascularization of the IVA with percutaneous angioplasty of other arterial targets. These techniques are certainly promising for the future, enriching the spectrum of surgery and maintaining its interest, but facing difficulties such as the learning curve, operative volume and cost[200, 201].

3.6.2. Graft selection

This study revealed a mean of 2.6±0.8 distal anastomoses per patient, comparable to those reported in other studies[39, 42, 45, 47-50, 52, 53, 55-57, 118].

Eighty-one patients received at least one VSI exceeding the 52% of Mhiri et al. [56]. Despite its ease of use, the venous graft has limitations in terms of long-term patency, with 40-50% occlusions at 5 years [202]. This is mainly due to venous degeneration of the graft and atherosclerosis of the venous graft [203].

We systematically used AMIG as a graft, with 24% of patients benefiting from revascularization by double internal mammary bypass. Our results were similar to Ueki [118] and exceeding most reported rates [39, 48, 55-57, 118]. The right internal mammary artery was less used, despite a 5-year patency of 91.2% [202]. This artery can be used pedicled or as a free graft, mainly to reach coronary segments distal enough for a pedicled graft.

In the specific context of LV dysfunction, it is imperative to focus on the long-term preservation of graft durability by minimizing the risks of thrombosis and degeneration. Both processes could have serious consequences, including myocardial infarction or chronic ischemia, which could further aggravate LV dysfunction or trigger decompensation of chronic heart failure.

Thus, with the aim of improving long-term results for patients with left ventricular dysfunction, multiple arterial revascularization has developed, favoring above all the use of the two internal thoracic arteries, but also the radial and more rarely the gastroepiploic arteries (116, 118, 119). Several techniques such as arterial Y, sequential anastomoses, or composite grafts (radial artery over mammary artery) have also been developed to increase the number of distal anastomoses [204-207]. The efficacy of composite arterial grafts has been proven [205]but the use of saphenous veins as composite grafts has produced contradictory results [202, 203, 208-210]. Data from the SAVE RITA [211]showed no significant difference between the two graft types in terms of overall survival and MACCE. In our study, only one vein graft was Y-mounted on an AMIG and it degenerated.

In conclusion, although VSI has its limitations, it remains a frequently chosen option in CABG surgery. There are several reasons for this choice:

1. Multiple arterial revascularization is hampered by the risk of mediastinal infection when using both mammary arteries
2. The radial artery has specific characteristics, such as a tendency to spasticity, which requires pharmacological treatment. In addition, it must be used for lesions of over 90%. Endoscopic harvesting is preferable to minimize aesthetic impact.
3. Harvesting the gastroepiploic artery presents difficulties.
4. Arterial revascularization is technically more complex.

Ongoing efforts are being made to improve the quality of VSI and explore other options to improve long-term outcomes [203].

3.6.3. Impact of incomplete revascularization

In our study, only 53% of patients underwent complete myocardial revascularization. Two important factors predisposing to incomplete revascularization were identified: the presence of calcifications in the coronary arteries and the presence of tandem lesions on the anterior interventricular artery (AIA).

Tandem lesions are characterized by severe narrowings in close proximity on the same coronary vessel, sometimes requiring specific intervention, especially when distal narrowings remain. This configuration can make the procedure more complex and compromise graft patency. In extreme cases, it may even be necessary to forego bypass surgery because of the severity of obstructions in downstream arteries.

The main aim of coronary bypass surgery is to bypass the lesions and perfuse the arteries downstream. However, surgery on heavily calcified arteries is not recommended, as it increases the risk of post-operative failure. Although coronary endarterectomy techniques exist to treat calcifications, they are often associated with disappointing results and an increased risk of thrombosis after the operation. It is essential to note that these predictive factors may coexist, further complicating revascularization[198]

Identifying and addressing these predictive factors is of crucial importance in improving surgical outcomes in patients with coronary artery disease and reduced LVEF, in order to avoid surgical interventions that may not offer significant advantages over percutaneous angioplasty. To optimize revascularization in these patients and improve their quality of life after surgery, innovative approaches and detailed planning are imperative.

By doing so, we can avoid committing these patients to potentially risky surgical procedures, preferring less invasive alternatives such as percutaneous angioplasty where appropriate. Ultimately, the main objective remains to improve the quality of life of patients with coronary artery disease and reduced LVEF, by choosing the best treatment strategy adapted to each individual case.

3.6.4. **Extracorporeal circulation and intraoperative circulatory assistance :**

Comparing our data with those in the literature, as illustrated in Table 23, we found some consistency with results reported in other studies. We identified prolonged CEC as a predictor of postoperative infections and delayed extubation. These two factors were also found to be predictive of MACCE. Moreover, postoperative infection is itself predictive of deterioration in LVEF fraction. Furthermore, postoperative infection and LVEF deterioration have been identified as predictors of early mortality.

These results underline the importance of rigorous monitoring of the duration of CEC and aortic clamping. Prolongation of these periods may be associated with an increased risk of postoperative complications, including infections and organ dysfunction. Particular attention should be paid to patients requiring prolonged circulatory assistance or the use of extracorporeal circulation devices (BCPIA), as these patients potentially present a higher risk of complications and mortality.

Table 23 Assessment of the duration of hemodynamic support based on studies in the literature.

Study	Duration CEC minutes	CLAO minutes	BCPIA Postop %	Intubation time Hours
Arom**[41]**	-	-	2,3	33,2±118,6
Mickleborough**[157]**	117,4± 30,7	69,5±17,9	15	-
Shennib**[42]**	91,5±42,2	62,2±19,1	6,5	16.5± 22.4
Ascione**[43]**	-	-	12	-
Hillis**[44]**	88	50		-
Darwazah**[45]**	107.4 ± 29.7	53.7±14.1		-
Filsoufi**[48]**	125 ±40	98± 50	11,9	-
Youn**[49]**	114.5±37.3	89.4±27.4		19.4±12.5
Caputti **[51]**			4,5	22,3
Emmert **[62]**	109±40	53±28	2,5	-
Keeling**[53]**	100.7±36.4	69.8± 28.2	-	-
Ueki**[118]**	153.5±59.1		-	-
MHIRI thesis **[56]**	75,3±25,5	49,2±15,1	-	8,4±15,6
Tribak **[57]**	132 ± 50	62 ± 19	14	-
Our study	**124±46,5**	**80,1±27,5**	**15**	**6±3**

4. Surgery results

4.1. Postoperative morbidity early

4.2. Major cardiovascular events

Table 24 compares the incidence rates of the main complications noted in the series with those in the literature.

Table 24: Analysis of early postoperative complications in the literature

STUDY	IDM	TAMPONNADE	FA	TV/FV	BAV	MÉDIASTINITE	INFECTION	IRA	HEMORRAGY	TIA/STROKE	SBDC
Arom K.V. [41]	NP	2,3	23	NP	NP	0	NP	NP	3,8	2,3	
Shennib H [42]	4,3	NP	10,9	8,7	NP	NP	10,9	NP	NP	4,3	8,7
Ascione R. [43]	NP	NP	21	4	3	9	NP	5	6	2	
Darwazah [45]	2,4	NP	4,8	8,3	NP	NP	7,1	7,1	9,5	1,2	9,5
Sharoni E. [46]	1	NP	1	NP	NP	NP	NP	5	1	1	
Wu et al [47]	1,6	NP	NP	2,7	NP	1,4	NP	1,6	0,8	1,6	3,3
Filsoufi	1	NP	NP	NP	NP	1	3	1	NP	NP	NP

STUDY	IDM	TAMPONNADE	FA	TV/FV	BAV	MÉDIASTINITE	INFECTION	IRA	HEMORRAGY	TIA/STROKE	SBDC
F. **[48]**											
Youn T.N. **[49]**	3,8	NP	NP	1	NP	NP	NP	NP	3,8	3,8	NP
Attaran S. **[50]**	3,8	NP	29,6	NP	NP	5,7	NP	9,3	4	2,3	NP
Caputti G.M. **[51]**	2,7	NP	NP	NP	NP	NP	10,7	8,7	NP	2,7	8
Emmert M.Y. **[52]**	3,2	0,2	4,2	NP	NP	NP	NP	6,3	6,7	2,3	4,1
Keeling W.B. **[53]**	0,7	NP	22,3	NP	NP	NP	NP	5,8	2,8	1,9	NP
Ueki C. **[118]**	0,6	NP	12,6	NP	NP	3,4	2,2	7,1	3,4	NP	NP

STUDY	IDM	TAMPONNADE	FA	TV/FV	BAV	MÉDIASTINITE	INFECTION	IRA	HEMORRAGY	TIA/STROKE	SBDC
Wang **[55]**	2,2	NP	NP	6,8	NP	2,2	4,5	NP	NP	4,5	2,2
MHIRI F. **[56]**	2,4	NP	4,8	NP	NP	2,3	9,5	17	2,3	0	
Tribak M. **[57]**	1,7	NP	NP	NP	NP	4,6	11,6	NP	4	2,9	10,5
Our study	2,7	2	4,1	1,3	2,7	4,1	28	19,4	1,3	1	37

TIA: Transient ischemic attack, **CVA:** Stroke, **AVB:** Atrioventricular block, **AF**: Atrial fibrillation, **VF:** Ventricular fibrillation, **HTA:** Hypertension, **MI:** Myocardial infarction**, ARF:** Acute renal failure, **SBDC:** Low cardiac output syndrome**, VT:** Ventricular tachycardia.

4.2.1.1. Acute coronary syndromes

Sixteen percent of patients had postoperative coronary events, including 7.2% NSTEMI and 2.7% STEMI. Of these, only 25% underwent post-operative angiographic monitoring. Comparing these results with those in the literature, the postoperative STEMI rate ranged from 0.6% in the STS registry[53] and 3.4% in the series by Shennib et al. [42]. Our prevalences of NSTEMI and STEMI were higher than those of the Moroccan series by Tribak et al. [57]who reported rates of 5.8% and 1.7% respectively. However, on a national scale, our results were consistent with those of Mhiri et al. [56]who reported prevalences of 7.1% and 2.4% respectively.

In our study, immediate postoperative myocardial infarction was a risk factor for early postoperative LVEF impairment.

Post-operative myocardial infarction is a recognized factor in post CABG morbidity and mortality. Its prevalence was 2-10% at the beginning of the CABG era [179, 212]. It may be linked to graft dysfunction, surgical technique, a poor downstream bed or a combination of these factors.
As for the graft, it may be of poor quality (small, pathological), have lesions associated with harvesting (haematoma, dissection) or present an anomaly in its course during deployment (torsion, hyperextension, spasm). Anastomotic malfunctions may be precipitated by the quality of the artery at the anastomosis site, but may also be inherent to the technique.
Factors inherent in the native circulation include inadequate myocardial protection, incomplete revascularization, and coronary embolization [213].

4.2.1.2. Stroke e

Only one patient had an early postoperative stroke, representing a prevalence of 1.3%. This rate is relatively low compared with the results of other previous research, which has shown post-PAC stroke rates ranging from 1% to 4.5% [48].

4.2.1.3. Acute heart failure and postoperative low cardiac output syndrome

SBDC represents the most frequent and severe complication following cardiac surgery. It is associated with a significant increase in short- and medium-term morbidity and mortality, as well as significant use of healthcare resources. Common complications associated with SBDC include acute renal failure, neurological problems, pulmonary complications and atrial fibrillation [214].

The results obtained are in line with those reported in the literature. Indeed, previously documented risk factors associated with SBDC include advanced age (greater than 65 years), female gender, presence of diabetes, tritruncal involvement, reduced LVEF, previous surgical procedures, recent myocardial infarction, incomplete revascularization, prolonged duration of CEC and ineffective intraoperative myocardial protection [215].
Treatment of SBDC is complex, with the aim of preventing further organ dysfunction and failure by providing appropriate hemodynamic support. If a cause is identified, it must be rapidly corrected. The first therapeutic step in SBDC, to be undertaken as soon as volume

status is optimized, is based on the use of inotropes and vasodilators to improve contractility, preload and afterload. Nevertheless, inotropic agents, mainly used in SBDC patients, can also improve cardiac output, but they achieve this goal at the cost of increased myocardial consumption and increased mortality risk [216]. Maintaining acid-base balance and normothermia, correcting electrolyte abnormalities and managing ventilation improve SBDC treatment outcomes and increase responsiveness to catecholamines [214].

The role of Levosimendan in the early postoperative phase is open to debate. It appears to reduce the risk of SBDC in some post-PAC patients with reduced LV function [217]. According to Eriksson et al. [218]Levosimendan improves cardiac output and facilitates weaning from bypass surgery. Tritapepe et al. [219] observed a significant drop in troponin levels after the use of Levosimendan in bypass surgery. Levin et al. [220] reported a reduced need for inotropes and vasopressors in patients treated with this drug. Van Diepen [221] noted a reduction in mechanical circulatory support at 5 days and in mortality rates at 30 and 90 days in the Levosimendan group compared with the placebo group.

However, the "LEVO-CTS" trial [169] on 882 patients with LV function≤ 35% found no significant difference in early morbidity between groups, although 90-day mortality was reduced in the Levosimendan group.

4.3. Early postoperative major non-cardiovascular complications

4.3.1.1. Bleeding complications

Bleeding and blood transfusions are frequent surgical complications in patients undergoing CABG.[222]. Abundant bleeding or sudden onset of bleeding is an indication for repeat surgery, irrespective of hemodynamic impact.

In this study, we observed a rebleeding rate of only 1.3%. These results are among the lowest in the literature, where rebleeding rates generally range from 1% to 9.5%. On a national scale, our rate was very close to that of the Sfax University Hospital, which was 2.3%.

Of the patients included, 2% required pericardiocentesis. This prevalence is similar to that reported by Arom K.V. et al.[41] in their own study. However, more recent studies have shown that this rate no longer exceeds 2‰ [62].

The mean postoperative deglobulation was 3.6±1.6 g/dl, and the median postoperative transfusion was two RGCs. These results are consistent with those reported by Ascione R. et al.[43].

Finally, in this reduced LVEF cohort with CABG, deglobulation with a postoperative Hb ≤ 9 g/dl was predictive of early mortality .

The need for further intervention to control bleeding occurs in two to six percent of CABG cases, and is accompanied by a 4.5-fold increase in mortality risk [223, 224]. Risk factors for postoperative bleeding and transfusion include advanced age, female gender, low body weight, preoperative cardiogenic shock, anemia, renal failure (particularly in patients on dialysis), peripheral vascular disease, poor nutritional status, recent thrombolytic therapy, unscheduled procedures, reoperations and prolonged bypass surgery. [224, 225].

4.3.1.2. Rhythmic complications

Postoperative AF occurred in some patients. This complication, although frequent with rates as high as 30% in the literature, had a lower prevalence of 4.1% in this study [226, 227].

Generally transient, this AF resolves in most patients within 2-3 days of treatment. However, patients with preoperative AF have shown little chance of spontaneous recovery of sinus rhythm. The origin of this complication is thought to be due to a series of factors, including pericardial inflammation, excessive catecholamine production and various neuro-hormonal imbalances postoperative [228-230]. This complication increases stroke risk, hospital stay, healthcare costs and mortality by two to three times [226, 231].

With regard to ventricular rhythm disorders, 1.3% presented with ventricular tachycardia. This rate was comparable to those reported in the literature. A study by Sadr-Ameli [232] on 856 patients undergoing coronary bypass surgery showed a 26.6% incidence of ventricular rhythm disorders, including 17.6% monomorphic nonsustained ventricular tachycardias, 5.4% monomorphic sustained ventricular tachycardias, 0.8% polymorphic ventricular tachycardias and 2.7% ventricular fibrillations. According to this study, preoperative LV dysfunction was a major predictor of ventricular rhythm disturbances postoperatively, along with other factors namely postoperative myocardial infarction or hemodynamic instability [232].

4.3.1.3. Infectious complications

The infectious complication was identified as an independent risk factor associated with increased short- and long-term morbidity and mortality. In addition, it has been shown to be a risk factor for postoperative deterioration in LVEF, the development of ARF, and prolongation of postoperative mechanical ventilation.

Early postoperative acute mediastinitis is a known complication after cardiac surgery with vertical median sternotomy, with an incidence ranging from 0.14 to 2.9% in studies, and up to 10% in some extreme cases [233, 234]. This complication tends to occur more frequently in coronary surgery than in valvular or combined procedures[234]. In our study, the prevalence of mediastinitis was 4.1%, whereas in the study by Mhiri et al. it was 6.9%.

Post-intubation bronchopulmonary infection was the most frequent complication, with a prevalence of 28%, exceeding the rates reported in the literature, which did not exceed 12%.

4.3.1.4. Acute renal failure

Nineteen percent developed acute renal failure early postoperatively. There was no correlation between the severity of pre-existing renal disease and postoperative worsening of renal function. However, the absence of pre-existing chronic kidney disease was identified as an indicator of a low risk of postoperative worsening.

In the literature, renal failure, integrated into the Euroscore II parameters, has been clearly established as a predictive factor of mortality by different teams, making it a major complication in patients undergoing cardiac surgery [235]. Its incidence can be as high as 39% in patients undergoing cardiac surgery[236]. Predictive factors for postoperative renal dysfunction have been described, including age, female gender, preoperative renal function[165, 237-242]duration of CEC, duration of aortic clamping, length of ICU stay and postoperative use of norepinephrine[165, 237-242]. In our study, the predictive factors of postoperative renal dysfunction were: postoperative SBDC, occurrence of an infectious complication, LVEF <38%, BMI>25 kg/m^2 ($p< 10^{-3}$), STS score risk>1.08%

and prolonged ventilation beyond 72 hours with good sensitivity and specificity for the latter .

Risk factors associated with acute renal failure in the context of cardiac surgery can be classified according to patient characteristics, the operative context and the nature of the surgical procedure.

Among patient-related risk factors, age [165, 237-242] as well as the presence of pre-existing CKD have been identified as determinants in international studies [165, 237-242]. However, the present study was unable to confirm these associations due to our small sample size, which is one of its limitations.

Regarding the clinical context, the urgency of surgery[238, 243-245]particularly if scheduled less than 24 hours after coronary angiography [243]has been associated with an increased risk of postoperative acute renal failure. The presence of hemodynamic instability[243, 245] and the use of mechanical circulatory support, such as an intra-aortic balloon, prior to surgery[238, 245]have been reported as risk factors in the literature.

With regard to procedure-related factors, a prolonged duration of extracorporeal circulation[246, 247] was associated with an increased risk of postoperative acute renal failure. It is possible that avoidance of bypass for and use of beating-heart CABG may be associated with a lower risk of acute renal failure [238, 248, 249].

4.3.1.1. Use of prolonged mechanical ventilation

Prolonged mechanical ventilation exceeding 72 hours was associated with increased morbidity and mortality in patients with LV systolic dysfunction or respiratory failure (158). Prolonged mechanical ventilation exposes patients to potential complications, such as mechanical ventilation-associated pneumonia, atelectasis, abdominal distension, stress ulcer and ventilation myopathy (158, 159).

In this study, the predictive factors for prolonged mechanical ventilation were: SBDC, postoperative infection and postoperative LVEF impairment.

4.3.2. Predictors of early major cardiovascular events

This study identified significant predictive factors for MACCE. These included postoperative infection, chronic renal failure, Euroscore II, STS score, prolonged mechanical ventilation and LVEF <33%.

These results provide essential information on postoperative complications, enabling the identification of patients at high risk of MACCE. Certain complications, such as healthcare-associated infections, showed higher prevalence rates than those reported in the literature, underlining the need for increased vigilance and reinforced preventive measures.

4.4. Postoperative evolution of left ventricular systolic ejection fraction

The evolution of left ventricular ejection fraction (LVEF) over the first month revealed that 36% of patients experienced an improvement in their LVEF, while 34% maintained a stable LVEF and 19% showed a deterioration. These results are consistent with those observed in other studies, notably that conducted by Elefteriades et al. [40]where an improvement of 36% was observed, as well as the study by Kron et al. [44] which reported a 42% improvement. In addition, Mhiri et al.[56] also found an early improvement in LVEF in 42% of patients.

Factors predictive of postoperative LVEF deterioration were: preoperative damage to the anterior and anteroseptal walls of the LV or incomplete revascularization, mainly of the IVA artery. Conversely, failure of complete revascularization of multiple marginal lesions or of the DC had no statistically significant relationship with early LVEF deterioration.

In addition, two postoperative complications were identified as being predictive of this early deterioration in LVEF. These were postoperative myocardial infarction and infection. No statistically significant relationship was found between LVEF decline and postoperative right ventricular longitudinal systolic function, duration of bypass surgery, duration of aortic clamping or duration of cardiac assistance.

This group showed a higher morbi-mortality with an increased incidence of postoperative acute renal failure and postoperative SBDC.

On the other hand, improvement in left ventricular ejection fraction (LVEF) during follow-up proved to be the only protective factor against the occurrence of major cardiovascular complications (MACCE) in the long term. These results confirm previous observations, in which preoperative left ventricular function was a predictor of both short- and long-term favorable outcomes after coronary revascularization surgery [36, 143].

International studies [125, 250-252] have demonstrated that coronary artery bypass graft surgery can increase LVEF by 5% to 18% in patients with myocardium in a state of sideration or hibernation. This improvement was often observed as early as the first few weeks after surgery and could persist for up to 10 years in some series, provided no cardiovascular complications occurred during this period[253, 254].

For example, in a study by Bax et al. [255]a 61% improvement in contractility of siderated myocardium was observed at three months after CABG, reaching 70% improvement at 14 months. In hibernating myocardium, contractility improved by 31% at three months and by 61% at 14 months.

With regard to preoperative assessment of myocardial viability, the same study [255] revealed that the presence of at least four viable segments per patient was directly associated with improved LVEF after revascularization. A threshold of four or more viable segments offered the highest sensitivity and specificity (86% and 92%, respectively) for predicting LVEF improvement. Moreover, the presence of four or more viable segments predicted an improvement in heart failure symptoms after revascularization, with positive and negative predictive values of 76% and 71%, respectively.

Finally, it should be noted that lack of improvement or progressive deterioration of LVEF in patients with siderated or hibernating myocardium after CABG surgery was generally associated with incomplete revascularization or graft occlusion[255].

4.1. Predictors of late major cardiovascular events

Chronic kidney disease (CKD) and the occurrence of postoperative infection have been shown to be predictors of both early and late major cardiovascular complications (MACCE). However, other factors were identified as predictors of late cardiovascular events only. Specifically, the use of extremely urgent coronary artery bypass graft (CABG) surgery after recent myocardial infarction, especially if complicated by acute heart failure or affecting anterior interventricular artery (AIV)-dependent myocardial mass. These results are in line with the literature, as previously demonstrated.

4.2. Survival studies:

Overall survival was estimated at 68.5% at 2 years and 57.9% at 5 years for the entire cohort.

In the literature, preoperative LVEF impairment has been identified as a very powerful predictor of intraoperative and 30-day mortality, hence its inclusion in surgical risk calculation scores [22, 133].

The mortality rate after CABG in patients with reduced LVEF varies according to the preoperative LVEF threshold adopted. Early mortality rates ranged from 0.8% to 11%. It was 5% to 11% for LVEF <20% [48, 256]2.1% to 11% for LVEF < 30%. [36, 257]4% to 10.5% for LVEF < 35%. [139, 258]1.6% to 6.7% for LVEF < 40% [125, 259]and 0.8% to 4.9% for LVEF < 50%. [125, 139, 259, 260].

A reduction in preoperative LVEF also influences long-term survival. Indeed, a reduced LVEF doubles the risk of cardiac death at 5 years [261].

Certain factors influenced survival and the occurrence of major cardiovascular events, including deterioration in LVEF, chronic renal failure, extreme emergency surgery and the onset of postoperative infection. In addition, statistically significant differences in the period free of major cardiovascular events as a function of LVEF changes during follow-up.

The presence of other risk factors can amplify the impact of reduced LVEF on postoperative morbidity and mortality. Elements such as advanced age, female gender, advanced NYHA class, left coronary artery stenosis, renal dysfunction, low hemoglobin and complexity of coronary disease have been associated with less favorable outcomes after CABG in these patients[38]

Each of these elements underscores the importance of careful preoperative and postoperative management to improve outcomes after CABG.

Despite the increased risk, CABG remains a viable option for carefully selected patients with reduced LVEF. With appropriate management peri-operatively, but especially pre-operatively (including optimal medical treatment of heart failure, control of cardiovascular risk factors and comorbidities) and collegial discussion within a multidisciplinary team (Heart Team), particularly for patients with viable myocardium, the results of surgical revascularization can be successful, even in patients with severely reduced LVEF.

Conclusions

The decision to undergo coronary artery bypass grafting (CABG) is based on a number of criteria, including the clinical context, systolic ventricular function, ischemic load and coronary anatomy. Particularly in the presence of complex factors such as tritruncal involvement with high SYNTAX score, left ventricular dysfunction or large areas of ischemia [31].

In recent years, the number of patients with reduced left ventricular ejection fraction (LVEF) who are candidates for CABG has increased. Indeed, unlike percutaneous angioplasty, studies have shown that CABG is superior to medical treatment alone, improving symptoms and increasing survival [34, 35]. Advances in perioperative management, surgical techniques and myocardial protection methods have encouraged practitioners to consider this option more frequently [36].

However, despite these improvements, the risk of surgery persists and could lead to increased morbidity and mortality.

In this context, identifying factors predictive of morbidity and mortality is of paramount importance in determining which individuals will benefit most from surgical revascularization procedures.

The aim of this study was to investigate the early and medium-term mortality of surgical myocardial revascularization under extracorporeal circulation (ECC) in patients with reduced LVEF (preoperative LVEF≤ 40%).

We conducted a retrospective, single-center study in collaboration between the cardiology and thoracic surgery departments of HMPIT over a ten-year period from January 2012 to December 2021 and including 73 patients undergoing coronary artery bypass graft surgery and having preoperative left ventricular dysfunction with LVEF ≤ 40%. Concomitant prior heart or valve surgery and those treating a mechanical complication of MI were not included. Incomplete records, lost to follow-up and beating heart surgeries were excluded.

For each patient, we collected demographic data, pre-, intra- and postoperative characteristics, early (≤ 30 days) and late postoperative complications, as well as survival, functional status and distant ultrasound data. The median duration of follow-up in our study was 8 years, with a minimum duration of one year and a maximum duration of 11 years.

The mean age of the patients studied was 60.5 ± 7.5 years (35 to 80 years), with a male predominance. The main cardiovascular risk factors were smoking (69%), type 2 diabetes (55%), overweight (53%) and hypertension (47%). In addition, 58% of patients had at least three cumulative cardiovascular risk factors.

With regard to comorbidities, 25% of patients had carotid stenosis, 14% had symptomatic chronic obliterative arteritis of the lower limbs (COAAL), 16% of patients had preoperative anemia, 95% of diabetics had poorly controlled diabetes and 23% of patients had chronic renal failure.

In terms of coronary disease, 35% of patients had a previous history of coronary disease, and 21% had undergone stent implantation. In 80% of cases, the indication for CABG followed an acute coronary syndrome (ACS), including 48% with non-ST-segment elevation myocardial infarction (NSTEMI) and 29% with persistent segment elevation myocardial infarction (STEMI). In addition, 27% of patients had preoperative signs of acute congestive heart failure (CHF).

Coronary angiography revealed tritruncular involvement in 82% of cases, bi-truncular in 16%; tight left common trunk (LCT) stenosis was observed in 27% of patients, 34% had at least one chronic total occlusion (CTO) and 10% had a tandem multi-stenotic anterior interventricular artery (IVA). In addition, 19% of patients had calcified lesions, 10% had multiple marginal lesions and 3% had a small marginal network.

At transthoracic echocardiography, mean LVEF was 37 ±3% (25 to 40%), of which 35% had LVEF ≤ 35%. Segmental kinetic disturbances were noted in all patients with 10% severe hypokinesia, 48% myocardial akinesia, one percent dyskinesia. Preoperative myocardial viability testing was performed in only 12% of patients.

Operatively, all patients had undergone arterial bypass through the left internal mammary artery (LMIMA) on the IVA, with an average of three distal anastomoses per patient. Complete revascularization was achieved in 53% of patients. The median duration of CEC was 119 minutes, and that of aortic clamping was 77 minutes. Weaning from CEC was easy in 59% of cases. Postoperative mechanical hemodynamic support with an aortic counterpulsation balloon (BCPIA) was required in 19% of patients.

The average time to extubation of patients after the end of the procedure was 6 ±3 hours (2 to 240 hours).

Postoperative ultrasound monitoring was performed in 89% of patients. Mean ejection fraction was 39.7 ±7.6% (range 20-54%). LVEF improved in 36% of patients, remained stable in 34% and decreased in 19%.

The main early postoperative cardiovascular events were early death (22%), postoperative low cardiac output syndrome (LCAS) (38%), postoperative acute coronary syndromes (16%) and stroke (1%).

After univariate analysis, the predictive factors for Early Mortality were :

- ✓ Comorbidities: History of chronic renal failure (CRF) or ACOMI
- ✓ Functional signs: The preoperative presence of NYHA III-IV exertional dyspnea.
- ✓ Anatomical factors: the presence of a tight TCG stenosis or multiple marginal lesions.
- ✓ Cardiovascular events: postoperative SBDC, postoperative myocardial infarction.
- ✓ Post-operative non-cardiovascular complications: acute renal failure, post-operative infection, use of mechanical ventilation for more than 10 hours.
- ✓ Postoperative echocardiographic factors: postoperative LVEF ≤ 33%.
- ✓ EuroSCORE II and STS risk scores had predictive thresholds for early mortality at 3.18% and 0.93%, respectively.

Among these factors, some were predictive of major cardiovascular events (MACCE), notably :

- ✓ A history of chronic renal failure.
- ✓ The occurrence of a postoperative infectious complication.
- ✓ Post-operative LVEF ≤33%.
- ✓ Use of mechanical ventilation for more than 9 hours.

The main predictors of early postoperative LVEF deterioration were:

- ✓ Disturbances in anteroseptal segmental kinetics preoperatively.
- ✓ Incomplete surgical revascularization of the IVA or circumflex artery (Cx) territory
- ✓ The occurrence of a postoperative infectious complication.

Of the 72 patients surviving after the hospital period, 50 were followed up.

Thirty-one patients (62%) were paucisymptomatic (NYHA stage II dyspnea) or asymptomatic. Twelve patients (24%) were symptomatic with stage III dyspnea, and 7 patients (14%) were symptomatic with stage IV dyspnea.

TTE at late follow-up showed that late left ventricular function improved in 24 patients (48%), was stable in 16 patients (32%), and was impaired in 10 patients (20%).

The median follow-up was 95 months (8 years), with extremes ranging from one month to 134 months (11 years).

Factors predictive of mortality during follow-up were :

- ✓ Extreme emergency surgery with clopidogrel.
- ✓ Disturbances in anteroseptal segmental kinetics (preoperative).
- ✓ Mediastinitis.
- ✓ Poorly controlled diabetes at the time of cardiac surgery.
- ✓ A drop in LVEF of at least 5%.

Factors predictive of MACCE during follow-up were:

- ✓ A history of chronic renal failure.
- ✓ Preoperative acute heart failure.
- ✓ Extreme emergency surgery without stopping clopidogrel.
- ✓ Disturbances in anteroseptal segmental kinetics preoperatively.
- ✓ The occurrence of a postoperative infectious complication.

Conversely, an improvement in LVEF ≥ 5% was associated with a better prognosis (OR= 0.2 (0.09; 0.8), p=0.049).

In multivariate analysis, the independent predictors of overall mortality were :

- ✓ The presence of kinetic disorders in the anterior or anteroseptal territory (OR=4.21; 95% CI (1; 15.77); p= 0.033).
- ✓ Extreme emergency surgery performed on clopidogrel (OR=1.1; 95% CI (1.45; 17.92); p= 0.011).
- ✓ Post-operative low cardiac output syndrome (OR=9.79; 95% CI (2.61; 36.75); p= 0.000 7).

Overall survival was estimated at 68.5% at 2 years and 57.9% at 5 years in the whole cohort according to the Kaplan Meyer model.

When LVEF stratification was taken into account, multivariate Cox regression revealed that early postoperative LVEF impairment, as well as during follow-up, were associated with an increased risk of mortality, with a Hazard Ratio (HR) of 3.62 and 5.44 respectively. Similarly, when considering LVEF stratification during follow-up, LVEF deterioration is associated with a higher risk of mortality, with an HR of 5.44.

MACCE-free survival was estimated at 60.3% at 2 years, and 43.8% at 5 years according to the Kaplan Meyer model.

Although surgery represents the "gold standard" of revascularization for tritruncular patients with diabetes or complex TCG involvement in addition to systolic left ventricular

dysfunction, it is associated with a non-negligible operative risk. This was reflected in the morbidity and mortality observed in our study.
The study of predictive factors makes it possible to assess risk, anticipate complications and optimize post-operative care.
Several predictive factors can be addressed prior to surgery, apart from emergency situations. This requires rigorous patient selection and a preoperative preparation phase, which is particularly important in view of co-morbidities such as diabetes and CKD, and in order to optimize the medical treatment of heart failure.
Although the operative data are not clear from our results, the time of aortic clamping and myocardial ischemia should be kept to a minimum, particularly to reduce the incidence of SBDC. Myocardial protection must be rigorous, whatever the strategy adopted. Several solutions exist, such as retrograde perfusion through the coronary sinus, either continuous or intermittent, or cardioplegia administration via bypass grafts, or a combination of several routes of administration without demonstrating superiority, and there is no consensus given the lack of studies with a high level of evidence. Beating-heart revascularization may represent a radical solution, avoiding aortic clamping and reducing the deleterious effects of bypass surgery, but it requires special logistics, a high level of expertise and a dedicated operating activity, given the added surgical complexity. The treatment of calcified and complex lesions and the approach to posterior lesions represent a major difficulty. These considerations are reflected in the recommendations of the European Society of Cardiology (ESC) and justify the IIa-B level of evidence for this practice.
Hybrid revascularization, combining percutaneous angioplasty and surgical myocardial revascularization, especially via a minimally invasive approach, may be of interest. It reduces surgical trauma and operating time, and does not require extracorporeal circulation. From a surgical point of view, the major limitations are the acquisition of suitable, expensive equipment, and expertise in minimally invasive surgery.
Over and above technical considerations, complete revascularization, preferably with arterial grafts, is a guarantee of long-term results and should be the preferred strategy, taking into account patient characteristics, the risk of complications at the surgical site, and the quality of the recipient axes.
The postoperative phase is critical in this population, and the high incidence of respiratory infectious complications had a major impact on morbidity and mortality. This is a major

challenge in the ICU for these high-risk patients, and rigorous strategies to limit these complications must be deployed.

Specific action on these predictive factors will help improve results, but prior to such action, a multidisciplinary heart team approach to the choice of therapeutic strategy is essential, taking into account patient characteristics and available resources.

However, these results must be interpreted taking into consideration certain limitations of our study:

- ✓ The relatively small sample size and monocentric nature of the study limit the statistical power and generalizability of the results to a larger population.
- ✓ The retrospective nature of the study, based on medical records, could lead to selection and information bias, affecting the accuracy of the results.
- ✓ Delays in data collection could influence results due to missing or incomplete data.
- ✓ The absence of a comparison group makes it difficult to specifically assess the impact of left ventricular systolic dysfunction on postoperative morbidity and mortality.
- ✓ Changes in clinical practices and medical advances since the study period may limit the relevance of current results.

Despite these limitations, the results of this study provide interesting insights into the predictors of morbidity and survival after surgical myocardial revascularization in cases of reduced LVEF. Further studies are needed to confirm and deepen our understanding of the clinical outcomes associated with this procedure.

References

References

1. Ralapanawa U, Sivakanesan R. Epidemiology and the Magnitude of Coronary Artery Disease and Acute Coronary Syndrome: A Narrative Review. J. Epidemiol. Glob. Health. 2021 Jun;11(2):169-77.

2. Neumann F-J, Sousa-Uva M, Ahlsson A, Alfonso F, Banning AP, Benedetto U, et al. 2018 ESC/EACTS Guidelines on myocardial revascularization. Eur. Heart J. 2018;40(2):87-165.

3. McDonagh TA, Metra M, Adamo M, Gardner RS, Baumbach A, Böhm M, et al. 2021 ESC Guidelines for the diagnosis and treatment of acute and chronic heart failure: Developed by the Task Force for the diagnosis and treatment of acute and chronic heart failure of the European Society of Cardiology (ESC) With the special contribution of the Heart Failure Association (HFA) of the ESC. Eur. Heart J. 2021;42(36):3599-726.

4. Seferovic PM, Vardas P, Jankowska EA, Maggioni AP, Timmis A, Milinkovic I, et al. The Heart Failure Association Atlas: Heart Failure Epidemiology and Management Statistics 2019. Eur. J. Heart Fail. 2021 Jun;23(6):906-14.

5. Charfeddine S, Yousfi C, Gtif I, Abid O, Sdiri W, Halima MB, et al. Epidemiology, management, and outcomes of heart failure in Tunisia: Results from the Nature-HF registry. Archives of Cardiovascular Diseases Supplements. 2020;12(1):45.

6. Abid L, Charfeddine S, Kammoun I, Ben Halima M, Ben Slima H, Drissa M, et al. Epidemiology of heart failure and long-term follow-up outcomes in a north-African population: Results from the NAtional TUnisian REgistry of Heart Failure (NATURE-HF). PLoS One. 2021;16(5):e0251658.

7. Gtif I, Bouzid F, Charfeddine S, Abid L, Kharrat N. Heart failure disease: An African perspective. Arch. Cardiovasc. Dis. 2021 Oct;114(10):680-90.

8. Hassanabad AF, MacQueen KT, Ali I. Surgical Treatment for Ischemic Heart Failure (STICH) trial: A review of outcomes. J. Card. Surg. 2019 Oct;34(10):1075-82.

9. Knuuti J, Wijns W, Saraste A, Capodanno D, Barbato E, Funck-Brentano C, et al. 2019 ESC Guidelines for the diagnosis and management of chronic coronary syndromes: the Task Force for the diagnosis and management of chronic coronary syndromes of the European Society of Cardiology (ESC). Eur. Heart J. 2020;41(3):407-77.

10. Otaki Y, Gransar H, Berman DS, Cheng VY, Dey D, Lin FY, et al. Impact of family history of coronary artery disease in young individuals (from the CONFIRM registry). Am. J. Cardiol. 2013 Apr 15;111(8):1081-6.

11. American Diabetes Association Professional Practice C. 2. Classification and Diagnosis of Diabetes: Standards of Medical Care in Diabetes-2022. Diabetes Care. 2022 Jan 1;45(Suppl 1):S17-S38.

12. Williams B, Mancia G, Spiering W, Agabiti Rosei E, Azizi M, Burnier M, et al. 2018 ESC/ESH Guidelines for the management of arterial hypertension. Eur. Heart J. 2018 Sep 1;39(33):3021-104.

13. Hedayatnia M, Asadi Z, Zare-Feyzabadi R, Yaghooti-Khorasani M, Ghazizadeh H, Ghaffarian-Zirak R, et al. Dyslipidemia and cardiovascular disease risk among the MASHAD study population. Lipids Health Dis. 2020 Mar 16;19(1):42.

14. James PT, Leach R, Kalamara E, Shayeghi M. The worldwide obesity epidemic. Obes. Res. 2001;9(S11):228S-33S.

15. Hardman RL, Jazaeri O, Yi J, Smith M, Gupta R, editors. Overview of classification systems in peripheral artery disease. Seminars in interventional radiology; 2014: Thieme Medical Publishers.

16. Donnan GA, Davis SM, Chambers BR, Gates PC. Surgery for prevention of stroke. Lancet. 1998 May 9;351(9113):1372-3.

17. Naylor AR, Ricco JB, de Borst GJ, Debus S, de Haro J, Halliday A, et al. Editor's Choice - Management of Atherosclerotic Carotid and Vertebral Artery Disease: 2017 Clinical Practice Guidelines of the European Society for Vascular Surgery (ESVS). Eur. J. Vasc. Endovasc. Surg. 2018 Jan;55(1):3-81.

18. Lindenfeld J. Prevalence of anemia and effects on mortality in patients with heart failure. Am. Heart J. 2005 Mar;149(3):391-401.

19. Levey AS, Eckardt KU, Tsukamoto Y, Levin A, Coresh J, Rossert J, et al. Definition and classification of chronic kidney disease: a position statement from Kidney Disease: Improving Global Outcomes (KDIGO). Kidney Int. 2005 Jun;67(6):2089-100.

20. Saffioti S, Burzotta F, Coluccia V, Trani C, Bruno P, Massetti M, Crea F. Usefulness of EuroSCORE systems for risk stratification. J. Cardiovasc. Med (Hagerstown). 2015 Feb;16(2):90-9.

21. Youn YN, Kwak YL, Yoo KJ. Can the EuroSCORE predict the early and mid-term mortality after off-pump coronary artery bypass grafting? Ann. Thorac. Surg. 2007 Jun;83(6):2111-7.

22. Nashef SA. The current role of EuroSCORE. Semin. Thorac. Cardiovasc. Surg. 2012 Spring;24(1):11-2.

23. Fisher JD. New York Heart Association Classification. Arch. Intern. Med. 1972 May;129(5):836.

24. Levey AS, Coresh J, Balk E, Kausz AT, Levin A, Steffes MW, et al. National Kidney Foundation practice guidelines for chronic kidney disease: evaluation, classification, and stratification. Ann. Intern. Med. 2003 Jul 15;139(2):137-47.

25. Lang RM, Badano LP, Mor-Avi V, Afilalo J, Armstrong A, Ernande L, et al. Recommendations for cardiac chamber quantification by echocardiography in adults: an update from the American Society of Echocardiography and the European Association of Cardiovascular Imaging. Eur. Heart J. Cardiovasc. Imaging. 2015 Mar;16(3):233-70.

26. Ryan TJ, Bauman WB, Kennedy JW, Kereiakes DJ, King SB, 3rd, McCallister BD, et al. Guidelines for percutaneous transluminal coronary angioplasty. A report of the American Heart Association/American College of Cardiology Task Force on Assessment of Diagnostic and Therapeutic Cardiovascular Procedures (Committee on Percutaneous Transluminal Coronary Angioplasty). Circulation. 1993 Dec;88(6):2987-3007.

27. Ybarra LF, Rinfret S, Brilakis ES, Karmpaliotis D, Azzalini L, Grantham JA, et al. Definitions and Clinical Trial Design Principles for Coronary Artery Chronic Total Occlusion Therapies: CTO-ARC Consensus Recommendations. Circulation. 2021 Feb 2;143(5):479-500.

28. Vassileva CM, Aranki S, Brennan JM, Kaneko T, He M, Gammie JS, et al. Evaluation of The Society of Thoracic Surgeons Online Risk Calculator for Assessment of Risk in Patients Presenting for Aortic Valve Replacement After Prior Coronary Artery Bypass Graft: An Analysis Using the STS Adult Cardiac Surgery Database. Ann. Thorac. Surg. 2015 Dec;100(6):2109-15; discussion 15-6.

29. Thygesen K, Alpert JS, Jaffe AS, Chaitman BR, Bax JJ, Morrow DA, et al. Fourth universal definition of myocardial infarction (2018). Eur. Heart J. 2019 Jan 14;40(3):237-69.

30. Schoonen A, van Klei WA, van Wolfswinkel L, van Loon K. Definitions of low cardiac output syndrome after cardiac surgery and their effect on the incidence of intraoperative LCOS: A literature review and cohort study. Front Cardiovasc Med. 2022;9:926957.

31. Loef BG, Epema AH, Navis G, Ebels T, Stegeman CA. Postoperative renal dysfunction and preoperative left ventricular dysfunction predispose patients to increased long-term mortality after coronary artery bypass graft surgery. Br. J. Anaesth. 2009 Jun;102(6):749-55.

32. Lam CS, Donal E, Kraigher-Krainer E, Vasan RS. Epidemiology and clinical course of heart failure with preserved ejection fraction. Eur. J. Heart Fail. 2011 Jan;13(1):18-28.

33. Haxhibeqiri-Karabdic I, Hasanovic A, Kabil E, Straus S. Improvement of ejection fraction after coronary artery bypass grafting surgery in patients with impaired left ventricular function. Med Arch. 2014 Oct;68(5):332-4.

34. Temporelli PL, Scapellato F, Corra U, Pistono M, Eleuteri E, Imparato A, Giannuzzi P. Perioperative and postoperative predictors of outcome in patients with low ejection fraction early after coronary artery bypass grafting: the additional value of left ventricular remodeling. Eur. J. Cardiovasc. Prev. Rehabil. 2008 Aug;15(4):441-7.

35. Wrobel K, Stevens SR, Jones RH, Selzman CH, Lamy A, Beaver TM, et al. Influence of baseline characteristics, operative conduct, and postoperative course on 30-day outcomes of coronary artery bypass grafting among patients with left ventricular dysfunction: results from the Surgical Treatment for Ischemic Heart Failure (STICH) trial. Circulation. 2015;132(8):720-30.

36. Salehi M, Bakhshandeh A, Rahmanian M, Saberi K, Kahrom M, Sobhanian K. Coronary Artery Bypass Grafting in Patients with Advanced Left Ventricular Dysfunction: Excellent Early Outcome with Improved Ejection Fraction. J.Tehran univ. heart cent. 2016 Jan 13;11(1):6-10.

37. Nardi F, Diena M, Caimmi PP, Iraghi G, Lazzero M, Cerin G, et al. Relationship between left atrial volume and atrial fibrillation following coronary artery bypass grafting. J. Card. Surg. 2012;27(1):128-35.

38. Soliman Hamad MA, van Straten AH, van Zundert AA, ter Woorst JF, Martens EJ, Penn OC. Preoperative prediction of early mortality in patients with low ejection fraction undergoing coronary artery bypass grafting. J. Card. Surg. 2011 Jan;26(1):9-15.

39. Kron IL, Flanagan TL, Blackbourne LH, Schroeder RA, Nolan SP. Coronary revascularization rather than cardiac transplantation for chronic ischemic cardiomyopathy. Ann. Surg. 1989 Sep;210(3):348-52; discussion 52-4.

40 Elefteriades JA, Tolis G, Jr, Levi E, Mills LK, Zaret BL. Coronary artery bypass grafting in severe left ventricular dysfunction: excellent survival with improved ejection fraction and functional state. J. Am. Coll. Cardiol. 1993 Nov 1;22(5):1411-7.

41. Arom KV, Flavin TF, Emery RW, Kshettry VR, Petersen RJ, Janey PA. Is low ejection fraction safe for off-pump coronary bypass operation? Ann. Thorac. Surg. 2000 Sep;70(3):1021-5.

42. Shennib H, Endo M, Benhamed O, Morin JF. Surgical revascularization in patients with poor left ventricular function: on- or off-pump? Ann. Thorac. Surg. 2002 Oct;74(4):S1344-7.

43. Ascione R, Narayan P, Rogers CA, Lim KH, Capoun R, Angelini GD. Early and midterm clinical outcome in patients with severe left ventricular dysfunction undergoing coronary artery surgery. Ann. Thorac. Surg. 2003 Sep;76(3):793-9.

44. Hillis GS, Zehr KJ, Williams AW, Schaff HV, Orzulak TA, Daly RC, et al. Outcome of patients with low ejection fraction undergoing coronary artery bypass grafting: renal function and mortality after 3.8 years. Circulation. 2006 Jul 4;114(1 Suppl):I414-9.

45. Darwazah AK, Abu Sham'a RA, Hussein E, Hawari MH, Ismail H. Myocardial revascularization in patients with low ejection fraction < or =35%: effect of pump technique on early morbidity and mortality. J. Card. Surg. 2006 Jan-Feb;21(1):22-7.

46. Sharoni E, Song HK, Peterson RJ, Guyton RA, Puskas JD. Off pump coronary artery bypass surgery for significant left ventricular dysfunction: safety, feasibility, and trends in methodology over time--an early experience. Heart. 2006 Apr;92(4):499-502.

47. Wu FY, Lu YC, Lai ST, Weng ZC, Huang CH. Coronary artery bypass grafting in patients with left ventricular dysfunction. J. Chin. Med. Assoc. 2006 May;69(5):218-23.

48. Filsoufi F, Rahmanian PB, Castillo JG, Chikwe J, Kini AS, Adams DH. Results and predictors of early and late outcome of coronary artery bypass grafting in patients with severely depressed left ventricular function. Ann. Thorac. Surg. 2007 Sep;84(3):808-16.

49. Youn YN, Chang BC, Hong YS, Kwak YL, Yoo KJ. Early and mid-term impacts of cardiopulmonary bypass on coronary artery bypass grafting in patients with poor left ventricular dysfunction: a propensity score analysis. Circ. J. 2007 Sep;71(9):1387-94.

50. Attaran S, Shaw M, Bond L, Pullan MD, Fabri BM. Does off-pump coronary artery revascularization improve the long-term survival in patients with ventricular dysfunction? Interact. Cardiovasc. Thorac. Surg. 2010 Oct;11(4):442-6.

51. Caputti GM, Palma JH, Gaia DF, Buffolo E. Off-pump coronary artery bypass surgery in selected patients is superior to the conventional approach for patients with severely depressed left ventricular function. Clinics (Sao Paulo). 2011;66(12):2049-53.

52. Emmert M, Salzberg S, Seifert B, Schurr U, Theusinger O, Hoerstrup S, et al. editors. Off-pump surgery is not a contraindication for patients with a severely decreased ejection fraction. Heart. Surg. Forum; 2011.

53. Keeling WB, Williams ML, Slaughter MS, Zhao Y, Puskas JD. Off-pump and on-pump coronary revascularization in patients with low ejection fraction: a report from the society of thoracic surgeons national database. Ann. Thorac. Surg. 2013 Jul;96(1):83-8: discussion 8-9.

54. Ueki C, Sakaguchi G, Akimoto T, Ohashi Y, Sato H. On-pump beating-heart technique is associated with lower morbidity and mortality following coronary artery bypass grafting: a meta-analysis. Eur. J. Cardiothorac. Surg. 2016 Nov;50(5):813-21.

55. Wang W, Wang Y, Piao H, Li B, Wang T, Li D, et al. Early and Medium Outcomes of On-Pump Beating-Heart versus Off-Pump CABG in Patients with Moderate Left Ventricular Dysfunction. Braz. J. Cardiovasc. Surg. 2019 Jan-Feb;34(1):62-9.

56. MHIRI F. Results of surgical myocardial revascularization in left ventricular dysfunction [Thesis: Medical Research thesis]. Sfax: University of Sfax; 2020.

57. Tribak M, Konate M, Saidi S, Mahfoudi L, Elhassani A, Leghlimi LH, et al. Coronary bypass surgery in patients with severe left ventricular systolic dysfunction: short- and long-term results. Ann. Cardiol. Angeiol (Paris). Feb 2022;71(1):11-6.

58. Emmert MY, Salzberg SP, Theusinger OM, Rodriguez H, Sundermann SH, Plass A, et al. Off-pump surgery for the poor ventricle? Heart Vessels. 2012 May;27(3):258-64.

59. Neumann F-J, Sousa-Uva M, Ahlsson A, Alfonso F, Banning A, Benedetto U, et al. 2018 ESC/EACTS Guidelines on myocardial revascularization. European heart journal. 2019;40(2):87-165.

60. Shah S, Benedetto U, Caputo M, Angelini GD, Vohra HA. Comparison of the survival between coronary artery bypass graft surgery versus percutaneous coronary intervention in patients with poor left ventricular function (ejection fraction <30%): a propensity-matched analysis. Eur. J. Cardiothorac. Surg. 2019 Feb 1;55(2):238-46.

61. Velazquez EJ, Lee KL, Jones RH, Al-Khalidi HR, Hill JA, Panza JA, et al. Coronary-Artery Bypass Surgery in Patients with Ischemic Cardiomyopathy. N. Engl. J. Med. 2016 Apr 21;374(16):1511-20.

62. Emmert MY, Salzberg SP, Seifert B, Rodriguez H, Plass A, Hoerstrup SP, et al. Is off-pump superior to conventional coronary artery bypass grafting in diabetic patients with multivessel disease? Eur. J. Cardiothorac. Surg. 2011 Jul;40(1):233-9.

63. Saito A, Motomura N, Miyata H, Takamoto S, Kyo S, Ono M, Japan Cardiovascular Surgery Database O. Age-specific risk stratification in 13488 isolated coronary artery bypass grafting procedures. Interact. Cardiovasc. Thorac. Surg. 2011 Apr;12(4):575-80.

64. Miśkowiec D, Walczak A, Ostrowski S, Wrona E, Bartczak K, Jaszewski R. Isolated coronary artery bypass grafting in extracorporeal circulation in patients over 65 years old - does age still matter? Kardiochir. Torakochirurgia Pol (Online). 2014 Jun;11(2):191-9.

65. Flather M, Rhee J-W, Boothroyd DB, Boersma E, Brooks MM, Carrié D, et al. The effect of age on outcomes of coronary artery bypass surgery compared with balloon angioplasty or bare-metal stent implantation among patients with multivessel coronary disease: a collaborative analysis of individual patient data from 10 randomized trials. J. Am. Coll. Cardiol. 2012;60(21):2150-7.

66. Naughton C, Feneck RO, Roxburgh J. Early and late predictors of mortality following on-pump coronary artery bypass graft surgery in the elderly as compared to a younger population. Eur. J. Cardiothorac. Surg. 2009;36(4):621-7.

67. Rocha AS, Pittella FJ, Lorenzo AR, Barzan V, Colafranceschi AS, Brito JO, et al. Age influences outcomes in 70-year or older patients undergoing isolated coronary artery bypass graft surgery. Rev. Bras. Cir. Cardiovasc. 2012 Jan-Mar;27(1):45-51.

68. Safaie N, Montazerghaem H, Jodati A, Maghamipour N. In-hospital complications of coronary artery bypass graft surgery in patients older than 70 years. J. cardiovasc. thorac. res. 2015;7(2):60.

69. Hassan A, Chiasson M, Buth K, Hirsch G. Women have worse long-term outcomes after coronary artery bypass grafting than men. The Canadian journal of cardiology. 2005;21(9):757-62.

70. Ahmed WA, Tully PJ, Knight JL, Baker RA. Female sex as an independent predictor of morbidity and survival after isolated coronary artery bypass grafting. The Annals of thoracic surgery. 2011;92(1):59-67.

71. Alam M, Bandeali SJ, Kayani WT, Ahmad W, Shahzad SA, Jneid H, et al. Comparison by meta-analysis of mortality after isolated coronary artery bypass grafting in women versus men. Am. J. Cardiol. 2013 Aug 1;112(3):309-17.

72. Ergunes K, Yilik L, Yetkin U, Lafci B, Bayrak S, Ozpak B, Gurbuz A. Early and Mid-term Outcomes in Female Patients Undergoing Isolated Conventional Coronary Surgery. J. cardiovasc. thorac. res. 2014;6(2):105-10.

73. Khan JK, Shahabuddin S, Khan S, Bano G, Hashmi S, Sami SA. Coronary artery bypass grafting in South Asian patients: Impact of gender. Ann Med Surg (Lond). 2016 Aug;9:33-7.

74. Koch CG, Khandwala F, Nussmeier N, Blackstone EH. Gender and outcomes after coronary artery bypass grafting: a propensity-matched comparison. J. Thorac. Cardiovasc. Surg. 2003 Dec;126(6):2032-43.

75. Cloin EC, Noyez L. Myocardial revascularisation in women: evaluation of hospital mortality and morbidity. Neth. Heart J. 2006 Feb;14(2):49-54.

76. Solimene MC. Coronary heart disease in women: a challenge for the 21st century. Clinics (Sao Paulo). 2010;65(1):99-106.

77. Clough RA, Leavitt BJ, Morton JR, Plume SK, Hernandez F, Nugent W, et al. The effect of comorbid illness on mortality outcomes in cardiac surgery. Arch. Surg. 2002 Apr;137(4):428-32; discussion 32-3.

78. Aronson S, Boisvert D, Lapp W. Isolated systolic hypertension is associated with adverse outcomes from coronary artery bypass grafting surgery. Anesth. Analg. 2002;94(5):1079-84.

79. Örki T, Adademir T, Aksüt M, Çevirme D, Kırali K, Alp M, Çakalağaoğlu KC. Factors associated with early mortality in haemodialysis patients undergoing coronary artery bypass surgery. Cardiovasc. J. Afr. 2017;28(2):108-11.

80. Kuduvalli M, Grayson AD, Oo AY, Fabri BM, Rashid A. The effect of obesity on mid-term survival following coronary artery bypass surgery. Eur. J. Cardiothorac. Surg. 2003 Mar;23(3):368-73.

81. Kunadian B, Dunning J, Millner RW. Modifiable risk factors remain significant causes of medium term mortality after first time Coronary artery bypass grafting. J. Cardiothorac. Surg. 2007 Dec 3;2(1):51.

82. Gürbüz HA, Durukan AB, Salman N, Uçar Hİ, Yorgancıoğlu C. Obesity is still a risk factor in coronary artery bypass surgery. Anadolu Kardiyol. Derg. 2014;14(7).

83. Devarajan J, Vydyanathan A, You J, Xu M, Sessler DI, Sabik JF, Bashour CA. The association between body mass index and outcome after coronary artery bypass grafting operations. Eur. J. Cardiothorac. Surg. 2016;50(2):344-9.

84. Terada T, Johnson JA, Norris C, Padwal R, Qiu W, Sharma AM, et al. Severe obesity is associated with increased risk of early complications and extended length of stay following coronary artery bypass grafting surgery. Journal of the American Heart Association. 2016;5(6):e003282.

85. Harvey R, Haluska B, Mundy J, Wood A, Griffin R, Shah P. Association between body mass index and outcome of coronary artery bypass. Asian Cardiovascular and Thoracic Annals. 2011;19(5):333-8.

86. Shahabuddin S, Perveen S, Furnaz S, Fatimi S, Sami S, Sharif H. Body mass index--predictor of outcome after coronary artery bypass grafting. Asian Cardiovasc. Thorac. Ann. 2013 Apr;21(2):176-80.

87. Ao H, Wang X, Xu F, Zheng Z, Chen M, Li L, et al. The impact of body mass index on short- and long-term outcomes in patients undergoing coronary artery graft bypass. PLoS One. 2014;9(4):e95223.

88. Furnaz S. Body Mass Index (BMI) as A Predictor of Outcome After Coronary Artery Bypass Grafting: An Asian Perspective. Value Health. 2014;17(7):A759.

89. van Straten AH, Hamad MAS, van Zundert AA, Martens EJ, Schönberger JP, de Wolf AM. Preoperative renal function as a predictor of survival after coronary artery bypass grafting: comparison with a matched general population. The journal of thoracic and cardiovascular surgery. 2009;138(4):971-6.

90. Romero-Corral A, Montori VM, Somers VK, Korinek J, Thomas RJ, Allison TG, et al. Association of bodyweight with total mortality and with cardiovascular events in coronary artery disease: a systematic review of cohort studies. Lancet. 2006 Aug 19;368(9536):666-78.

91. Le-Bert G, Santana O, Pineda AM, Zamora C, Lamas GA, Lamelas J. The obesity paradox in elderly obese patients undergoing coronary artery bypass surgery. Interact. Cardiovasc. Thorac. Surg. 2011 Aug;13(2):124-7.

92. Benedetto U, Danese C, Codispoti M. Obesity paradox in coronary artery bypass grafting: myth or reality? J. Thorac. Cardiovasc. Surg. 2014 May;147(5):1517-23.

93. Reeves BC, Ascione R, Chamberlain MH, Angelini GD. Effect of body mass index on early outcomes in patients undergoing coronary artery bypass surgery. J. Am. Coll. Cardiol. 2003 Aug 20;42(4):668-76.

94. Atalan N, Fazliogullari O, Kunt AT, Basaran C, Gurer O, Sitilci T, et al. Effect of body mass index on early morbidity and mortality after isolated coronary artery bypass graft surgery. J. Cardiothorac. Vasc. Anesth. 2012 Oct;26(5):813-7.

95. Nauffal V, Schwann TA, Yammine MB, El-Hage-Sleiman AK, El Zein MH, Kabour A, et al. Impact of prior intracoronary stenting on late outcomes of coronary artery bypass surgery in diabetics with triple-vessel disease. J. Thorac. Cardiovasc. Surg. 2015 May;149(5):1302-9.

96. Stevens LM, Khairy P, Agnihotri AK. Coronary artery bypass grafting after recent or remote percutaneous coronary intervention in the Commonwealth of Massachusetts. Circ. Cardiovasc. Interv. 2010 Oct;3(5):460-7.

97. Efird JT, O'Neal WT, O'Neal JB, Ferguson TB, Chitwood WR, Kypson AP. Effect of peripheral arterial disease and race on survival after coronary artery bypass grafting. Ann. Thorac. Surg. 2013 Jul;96(1):112-8.

98. Shay JW, Homma N, Zhou R, Naseer MI, Chaudhary AG, Al-Qahtani M, et al. Abstracts from the 3rd International Genomic Medicine Conference (3rd IGMC 2015) : Jeddah, Kingdom of Saudi Arabia. 30 November - 3 December 2015. BMC Genomics. 2016 Jul 20;17 Suppl 6(Suppl 6):487.

99. Roffi M, Ribichini F, Castriota F, Cremonesi A. Management of combined severe carotid and coronary artery disease. Curr. Cardiol. Rep. 2012 Apr;14(2):125-34.

100. da Rosa MP, Schwendler R, Lopes R, Portal VL. Carotid Artery Stenosis Associated with Increased Mortality in Patients who Underwent Coronary Artery Bypass Grafting: A Single Center Experience. Open Cardiovasc. Med. J. 2013;7:76-81.

101. Augoustides JG. Advances in the management of carotid artery disease: focus on recent evidence and guidelines. J. Cardiothorac. Vasc. Anesth. 2012 Feb;26(1):166-71.

102. Abid L, Hammami R, Chamtouri I, Drissa M, Boudiche S, Bahloul M, et al. Epidemiologic features and management of hypertension in Tunisia, the results from the Hypertension National Registry (NaTuRe HTN). BMC Cardiovasc. Disord. 2022 Mar 29;22(1):131.

103. Goursaud S, Du Cheyron D. Cardiorenal syndrome: diagnosis, pathophysiology and management. Intensive care medicine. 2014;23(6):585-94.

104. Jankowski J, Floege J, Fliser D, Bohm M, Marx N. Cardiovascular Disease in Chronic Kidney Disease: Pathophysiological Insights and Therapeutic Options. Circulation. 2021 Mar 16;143(11):1157-72.

105. Doenst T, Haddad H, Stebbins A, Hill JA, Velazquez EJ, Lee KL, et al. Renal Function and Coronary Bypass Surgery in Patients With Ischemic Heart Failure-Insights From the STICH Trial. Circulation. 2018;138(Suppl_1):A11902-A.

106. Minakata K, Bando K, Tanaka S, Takanashi S, Konishi H, Miyamoto Y, et al. Preoperative chronic kidney disease as a strong predictor of postoperative infection and mortality after coronary artery bypass grafting. Circ. J. 2014;78(9):2225-31.

107. Kalantar-Zadeh K, Jafar TH, Nitsch D, Neuen BL, Perkovic V. Chronic kidney disease. Lancet. 2021 Aug 28;398(10302):786-802.

108. Coresh J, Turin TC, Matsushita K, Sang Y, Ballew SH, Appel LJ, et al. Decline in estimated glomerular filtration rate and subsequent risk of end-stage renal disease and mortality. JAMA. 2014 Jun 25;311(24):2518-31.

109. Howell NJ, Keogh BE, Bonser RS, Graham TR, Mascaro J, Rooney SJ, et al. Mild renal dysfunction predicts in-hospital mortality and post-discharge survival following cardiac surgery. Eur. J. Cardiothorac. Surg. 2008 Aug;34(2):390-5; discussion 5.

110. Jayasekera H, Harvey R, Pinto N, Mundy J, Wood A, Beller E, et al. editors. Primary coronary artery bypass surgery in the presence of decreasing preoperative renal function: effect on short-term outcomes. Heart. Surg. Forum; 2012.

111. Holzmann MJ, Sartipy U. Relation between preoperative renal dysfunction and cardiovascular events (stroke, myocardial infarction, or heart failure or death) within three months of isolated coronary artery bypass grafting. The American journal of cardiology. 2013;112(9):1342-6.

112. O'Boyle F, Mediratta N, Chalmers J, Al-Rawi O, Mohan K, Shaw M, Poullis M. Long-term survival of patients with pulmonary disease undergoing coronary artery bypass surgery. Eur. J. Cardiothorac. Surg. 2013 Apr;43(4):697-703.

113. Ho PM, Arciniegas DB, Grigsby J, McCarthy M, Jr, McDonald GO, Moritz TE, et al. Predictors of cognitive decline following coronary artery bypass graft surgery. Ann. Thorac. Surg. 2004 Feb;77(2):597-603; discussion

114. Samuels LE, Kaufman MS, Morris RJ, Promisloff R, Brockman SK. Coronary artery bypass grafting in patients with COPD. Chest. 1998 Apr;113(4):878-82.

115. Bingol H, Cingoz F, Balkan A, Kilic S, Bolcal C, Demirkilic U, Tatar H. The effect of oral prednisolone with chronic obstructive pulmonary disease undergoing coronary artery bypass surgery. J. Card. Surg. 2005 May-Jun;20(3):252-6.

116. Leavitt BJ, Ross CS, Spence B, Surgenor SD, Olmstead EM, Clough RA, et al. Long-term survival of patients with chronic obstructive pulmonary disease undergoing coronary artery bypass surgery. Circulation. 2006 Jul 4;114(1 Suppl):I430-4.

117. Savas Oz B, Kaya E, Arslan G, Karabacak K, Cingoz F, Arslan M. Pre-treatment before coronary artery bypass surgery improves post-operative outcomes in moderate chronic obstructive pulmonary disease patients: cardiovascular topics. Cardiovasc. J. Afr. 2013;24(5):184-7.

118. Ueki C, Miyata H, Motomura N, Sakaguchi G, Akimoto T, Takamoto S. Off-pump versus on-pump coronary artery bypass grafting in patients with left ventricular dysfunction. J. Thorac. Cardiovasc. Surg. 2016 Apr;151(4):1092-8.

119. Nagendran J, Norris CM, Graham MM, Ross DB, Macarthur RG, Kieser TM, et al. Coronary revascularization for patients with severe left ventricular dysfunction. Ann. Thorac. Surg. 2013 Dec;96(6):2038-44.

120 Algarni KD, Elhenawy AM, Maganti M, Collins S, Yau TM. Decreasing prevalence but increasing importance of left ventricular dysfunction and reoperative surgery in prediction of mortality in coronary artery bypass surgery: trends over 18 years. J. Thorac. Cardiovasc. Surg. 2012 Aug;144(2):340-6, 6 e1.

121. Fukui T, Tabata M, Morita S, Takanashi S. Early and long-term outcomes of coronary artery bypass grafting in patients with acute coronary syndrome versus stable angina pectoris. J. Thorac. Cardiovasc. Surg. 2013 Jun;145(6):1577-83, 83 e1.

122. Dayan V, Soca G, Parma G, Mila R. Does early coronary artery bypass surgery improve survival in non-ST acute myocardial infarction? Interact. Cardiovasc. Thorac. Surg. 2013;17(1):140-2.

123. Nichols EL, McCullough JN, Ross CS, Kramer RS, Westbrook BM, Klemperer JD, et al. Optimal Timing From Myocardial Infarction to Coronary Artery Bypass Grafting on Hospital Mortality. Ann. Thorac. Surg. 2017 Jan;103(1):162-71.

124. Lang Q, Qin C, Meng W. Appropriate Timing of Coronary Artery Bypass Graft Surgery for Acute Myocardial Infarction Patients: A Meta-Analysis. Front Cardiovasc Med. 2022;9:794925.

125. Lorusso R, La Canna G, Ceconi C, Borghetti V, Totaro P, Parrinello G, et al. Long-term results of coronary artery bypass grafting procedure in the presence of left ventricular dysfunction and hibernating myocardium. Eur. J. Cardiothorac. Surg. 2001 Nov;20(5):937-48.

126. Nalla BP, Freedman J, Hare GM, Mazer CD. Update on blood conservation for cardiac surgery. J. Cardiothorac. Vasc. Anesth. 2012 Feb;26(1):117-33.

127. Rigal JC, Florence D, Marc A, Gaillard A, Betbeze V, Rozec B. Evaluation of transfusion rates for coronary artery bypass grafting (CABG) and aortic valve replacement (AVR) performed with bypass grafting, measurement of the impact of blood-sparing strategies. Transfus. Clin. Biol. Nov 2018;25(4):316.

128. Koch CG, Li L, Duncan AI, Mihaljevic T, Cosgrove DM, Loop FD, et al. Morbidity and mortality risk associated with red blood cell and blood-component transfusion in isolated coronary artery bypass grafting. Crit. Care Med. 2006 Jun;34(6):1608-16.

129. Paone G, Likosky DS, Brewer R, Theurer PF, Bell GF, Cogan CM, Prager RL. Transfusion of 1 and 2 units of red blood cells is associated with increased morbidity and mortality. The Annals of thoracic surgery. 2014;97(1):87-94.

130. Pagano D, Milojevic M, Meesters MI, Benedetto U, Bolliger D, von Heymann C, et al. 2017 EACTS/EACTA Guidelines on patient blood management for adult cardiac surgery. Eur. J. Cardiothorac. Surg. 2018 Jan 1;53(1):79-111.

131. Society of Thoracic Surgeons Blood Conservation Guideline Task F, Ferraris VA, Brown JR, Despotis GJ, Hammon JW, Reece TB, et al. 2011 update to the Society of Thoracic Surgeons and the Society of Cardiovascular Anesthesiologists blood conservation clinical practice guidelines. Ann. Thorac. Surg. 2011 Mar;91(3):944-82.

132. Agarwal GR, Krishna N, Raveendran G, Jose R, Padmanabhan M, Jayant A, Varma PK. Early outcomes in patients undergoing off-pump coronary artery bypass grafting. Indian J Thorac Cardiovasc Surg. 2019 Apr;35(2):168-74.

133. Shroyer AL, Grover FL, Hattler B, Collins JF, McDonald GO, Kozora E, et al. On-pump versus off-pump coronary-artery bypass surgery. N. Engl. J. Med. 2009 Nov 5;361(19):1827-37.

134. Tennyson C, Lee R, Attia R. Is there a role for HbA1c in predicting mortality and morbidity outcomes after coronary artery bypass graft surgery? Interact. Cardiovasc. Thorac. Surg. 2013;17(6):1000-8.

135. Munnee K, Bundhun PK, Quan H, Tang Z. Comparing the Clinical Outcomes Between Insulin-treated and Non-insulin-treated Patients With Type 2 Diabetes Mellitus After Coronary Artery Bypass Surgery: A Systematic Review and Meta-analysis. Medicine (Baltimore). 2016 Mar;95(10):e3006.

136. Strahan S, Harvey RM, Campbell-Lloyd A, Beller E, Mundy J, Shah P. Diabetic control and coronary artery bypass: effect on short-term outcomes. Asian Cardiovasc. Thorac. Ann. 2013 Jun;21(3):281-7.

137. Pang PY, Lim YP, Ong KK, Chua YL, Sin YK. 2015 Young Surgeon's Award Winner: Long-term Prognosis in Patients with Diabetes Mellitus after Coronary Artery Bypass Grafting: A Propensity-Matched Study. Ann. Acad. Med. Singapore. 2016 Mar;45(3):83-90.

138. Anesthetic Management For Enhanced Recovery After Cardiac Surgery (ERACS). In: Sofjan IP, McCutchan A. StatPearls [Internet]: StatPearls Publishing; 2022.

139. Soliman Hamad MA, van Straten AH, Schönberger JP, ter Woorst JF, de Wolf AM, Martens EJ, van Zundert AA. Preoperative ejection fraction as a predictor of survival after coronary artery bypass grafting: comparison with a matched general population. J. Cardiothorac. Surg. 2010;5(1):1-8.

140 Shroyer AL, Coombs LP, Peterson ED, Eiken MC, DeLong ER, Chen A, et al. The Society of Thoracic Surgeons: 30-day operative mortality and morbidity risk models. Ann. Thorac. Surg. 2003 Jun;75(6):1856-64; discussion 64-5.

141. Davoodi S, Karimi A, Ahmadi SH, Marzban M, Movahhedi N, Abbasi K, et al. Coronary artery bypass grafting in patients with low ejection fraction: the effect of intra-aortic balloon pump insertion on early outcome. Indian J. Med. Sci. 2008 Aug;62(8):314-22.

142. Ding W, Ji Q, Shi Y, Ma R. Predictors of low cardiac output syndrome after isolated coronary artery bypass grafting. Int. Heart J. 2015;56(2):144-9.

143. Gatti G, Maschietto L, Dell'Angela L, Benussi B, Forti G, Dreas L, et al. Predictors of immediate and long-term outcomes of coronary bypass surgery in patients with left ventricular dysfunction. Heart Vessels. 2016 Jul;31(7):1045-55.

144. Alderman EL, Bourassa MG, Cohen LS, Davis KB, Kaiser GG, Killip T, et al. Ten-year follow-up of survival and myocardial infarction in the randomized Coronary Artery Surgery Study. Circulation. 1990 Nov;82(5):1629-46.

145. Braunwald E, Kloner RA. The stunned myocardium: prolonged, postischemic ventricular dysfunction. Circulation. 1982 Dec;66(6):1146-9.

146. Ait Houssa M, Moutakiallah Y, Abdou A, Selkane C, Amahzoune B, Drissi M, et al. Results of coronary bypass surgery in left ventricular dysfunction (comparison of beating heart and bypass surgery). Ann. Cardiol. Angeiol (Paris). August 2013;62(4):241-7.

147. HATTACH L. Revascularization by coronary artery bypass grafting in patients with left ventricular dysfunction with ejection fraction ≤35% of ischemic origin [Thesis: Medical Research thesis]. Rabat: Mohammed V Univeristy; 2017.

148. Cortigiani L, Bigi R, Sicari R. Is viability still viable after the STICH trial? Eur. Heart J. Cardiovasc. Imaging. 2012 Mar;13(3):219-26.

149. Afridi I, Grayburn PA, Panza JA, Oh JK, Zoghbi WA, Marwick TH. Myocardial viability during dobutamine echocardiography predicts survival in patients with coronary artery disease and severe left ventricular systolic dysfunction. J. Am. Coll. Cardiol. 1998 Oct;32(4):921-6.

150. Senior R, Kaul S, Lahiri A. Myocardial viability on echocardiography predicts long-term survival after revascularization in patients with ischemic congestive heart failure. J. Am. Coll. Cardiol. 1999 Jun;33(7):1848-54.

151. Sawada S, Bapat A, Vaz D, Weksler J, Fineberg N, Greene A, et al. Incremental value of myocardial viability for prediction of long-term prognosis in surgically revascularized patients with left ventricular dysfunction. J. Am. Coll. Cardiol. 2003 Dec 17;42(12):2099-105.

152. Bax JJ, Poldermans D, Elhendy A, Cornel JH, Boersma E, Rambaldi R, et al. Improvement of left ventricular ejection fraction, heart failure symptoms and prognosis after revascularization in patients with chronic coronary artery disease and viable myocardium detected by dobutamine stress echocardiography. J. Am. Coll. Cardiol. 1999 Jul;34(1):163-9.

153. Chaudhry FA, Tauke JT, Alessandrini RS, Vardi G, Parker MA, Bonow RO. Prognostic implications of myocardial contractile reserve in patients with coronary artery disease and left ventricular dysfunction. J. Am. Coll. Cardiol. 1999 Sep;34(3):730-8.

154. Sicari R, Picano E, Cortigiani L, Borges AC, Varga A, Palagi C, et al. Prognostic value of myocardial viability recognized by low-dose dobutamine echocardiography in chronic ischemic left ventricular dysfunction. Am. J. Cardiol. 2003 Dec 1;92(11):1263-6.

155. Pasquet A, Robert A, D'Hondt AM, Dion R, Melin JA, Vanoverschelde JL. Prognostic value of myocardial ischemia and viability in patients with chronic left ventricular ischemic dysfunction. Circulation. 1999 Jul 13;100(2):141-8.

156. Karabulut A, Cakmak M. Treatment strategies in the left main coronary artery disease associated with acute coronary syndromes. J Saudi Heart Assoc. 2015 Oct;27(4):272-6.

157. Mickleborough LL, Carson S, Tamariz M, Ivanov J. Results of revascularization in patients with severe left ventricular dysfunction. J. Thorac. Cardiovasc. Surg. 2000 Mar;119(3):550-7.

158. Ertelt K, Genereux P, Mintz GS, Reiss GR, Kirtane AJ, Madhavan MV, et al. Impact of the severity of coronary artery calcification on clinical events in patients undergoing coronary artery bypass grafting (from the Acute Catheterization and Urgent Intervention Triage Strategy Trial). Am. J. Cardiol. 2013 Dec 1;112(11):1730-7.

159. Bourantas CV, Zhang YJ, Garg S, Mack M, Dawkins KD, Kappetein AP, et al. Prognostic implications of severe coronary calcification in patients undergoing coronary artery bypass surgery: an analysis of the SYNTAX study. Catheter. Cardiovasc. Interv. 2015 Feb 1;85(2):199-206.

160. Cao C, Indraratna P, Ang SC, Manganas C, Park J, Bannon PG, Yan TD. Should clopidogrel be discontinued before coronary artery bypass grafting for patients with acute coronary syndrome? A systematic review and meta-analysis. J. Thorac. Cardiovasc. Surg. 2014 Dec;148(6):3092-8.

161. Sorsa T, Pollesello P, Solaro RJ. The contractile apparatus as a target for drugs against heart failure: interaction of levosimendan, a calcium sensitiser, with cardiac troponin c. Mol. Cell. Biochem. 2004 Nov;266(1-2):87-107.

162. Paakkonen K, Annila A, Sorsa T, Pollesello P, Tilgmann C, Kilpelainen I, et al. Solution structure and main chain dynamics of the regulatory domain (Residues 1-91) of human cardiac troponin C. J. Biol. Chem. 1998 Jun 19;273(25):15633-8.

163 Endoh M. Mechanisms of action of novel cardiotonic agents. J. Cardiovasc. Pharmacol. 2002 Sep;40(3):323-38.

164. Tholen M, Ricksten SE, Lannemyr L. Effects of levosimendan on renal blood flow and glomerular filtration in patients with acute kidney injury after cardiac surgery: a double blind, randomized placebo-controlled study. Crit. Care. 2021 Jun 12;25(1):207.

165. Bove T, Calabro MG, Landoni G, Aletti G, Marino G, Crescenzi G, et al. The incidence and risk of acute renal failure after cardiac surgery. J. Cardiothorac. Vasc. Anesth. 2004 Aug;18(4):442-5.

166. Harrison RW, Hasselblad V, Mehta RH, Levin R, Harrington RA, Alexander JH. Effect of levosimendan on survival and adverse events after cardiac surgery: a meta-analysis. J. Cardiothorac. Vasc. Anesth. 2013 Dec;27(6):1224-32.

167. Cholley B, Caruba T, Grosjean S, Amour J, Ouattara A, Villacorta J, et al. Effect of Levosimendan on Low Cardiac Output Syndrome in Patients With Low Ejection Fraction Undergoing Coronary Artery Bypass Grafting With Cardiopulmonary Bypass: The LICORN Randomized Clinical Trial. JAMA. 2017 Aug 8;318(6):548-56.

168. Landoni G, Lomivorotov VV, Alvaro G, Lobreglio R, Pisano A, Guarracino F, et al. Levosimendan for Hemodynamic Support after Cardiac Surgery. N. Engl. J. Med. 2017 May 25;376(21):2021-31.

169. Mehta RH, Van Diepen S, Meza J, Bokesch P, Leimberger JD, Tourt-Uhlig S, et al. Levosimendan in patients with left ventricular systolic dysfunction undergoing cardiac surgery on cardiopulmonary bypass: Rationale and study design of the Levosimendan in Patients with Left Ventricular Systolic Dysfunction Undergoing Cardiac Surgery Requiring Cardiopulmonary Bypass (LEVO-CTS) trial. Am. Heart J. 2016 Dec;182:62-71.

170 Guarracino F, Heringlake M, Cholley B, Bettex D, Bouchez S, Lomivorotov VV, et al. Use of Levosimendan in Cardiac Surgery: An Update After the LEVO-CTS, CHEETAH, and LICORN Trials in the Light of Clinical Practice. J. Cardiovasc. Pharmacol. 2018 Jan;71(1):1-9.

171. Caruba T, Hourton D, Sabatier B, Rousseau D, Tibi A, Hoffart-Jourdain C, et al. Rationale and design of the multicenter randomized trial investigating the effects of levosimendan pretreatment in patients with low ejection fraction (≤ 40%) undergoing CABG with cardiopulmonary bypass (LICORN study). J. Cardiothorac. Surg. 2016;11:1-7.

172. Schiefenhovel F, Berger C, Penkova L, Grubitzsch H, Haller B, Meyer A, et al. Influence of timing of Levosimendan administration on outcomes in cardiac surgery. Front Cardiovasc Med. 2023;10:1213696.

173. Bouabdallaoui N, Stevens SR, Doenst T, Petrie MC, Al-Attar N, Ali IS, et al. Society of Thoracic Surgeons Risk Score and EuroSCORE-2 Appropriately Assess 30-Day Postoperative Mortality in the STICH Trial and a Contemporary Cohort of Patients With Left Ventricular Dysfunction Undergoing Surgical Revascularization. Circ. Heart Fail. 2018 Nov;11(11):e005531.

174. Maziak DE, Rao V, Christakis GT, Buth KJ, Sever J, Fremes SE, Goldman BS. Can patients with left main stenosis wait for coronary artery bypass grafting? Ann. Thorac. Surg. 1996 Feb;61(2):552-7.

175. da Rocha ASC, da Silva PRD. Can Patients with Left Main Coronary Artery Disease Wait for Myocardial Revascularization Surgery? Arq. Bras. Cardiol. 2003;80(2):191-3.

176 Melrose DG, Dreyer B, Bentall HH, Baker JB. Elective cardiac arrest. Lancet. 1955 Jul 2;269(6879):21-2.

177. Lillehei CW, Dewall RA, Gott VL, Varco RL. The direct vision correction of calcific aortic stenosis by means of a pump-oxygenator and retrograde coronary sinus perfusion. Dis. Chest. 1956 Aug;30(2):123-32.

178. Parolari A, Rubini P, Cannata A, Bonati L, Alamanni F, Tremoli E, Biglioli P. Endothelial damage during myocardial preservation and storage. Ann. Thorac. Surg. 2002 Feb;73(2):682-90.

179. Farkouh ME, Domanski M, Sleeper LA, Siami FS, Dangas G, Mack M, et al. Strategies for multivessel revascularization in patients with diabetes. N. Engl. J. Med. 2012 Dec 20;367(25):2375-84.

180. Ovrum E, Tangen G, Tollofsrud S, Oystese R, Ringdal MA, Istad R. Cold blood cardioplegia versus cold crystalloid cardioplegia: a prospective randomized study of 1440 patients undergoing coronary artery bypass grafting. J. Thorac. Cardiovasc. Surg. 2004 Dec;128(6):860-5.

181 Jacob S, Kallikourdis A, Sellke F, Dunning J. Is blood cardioplegia superior to crystalloid cardioplegia? Interact. Cardiovasc. Thorac. Surg. 2008 May;7(3):491-8.

182. Guru V, Omura J, Alghamdi AA, Weisel R, Fremes SE. Is blood superior to crystalloid cardioplegia? A meta-analysis of randomized clinical trials. Circulation. 2006 Jul 4;114(1 Suppl):I331-8.

183. Zeng J, He W, Qu Z, Tang Y, Zhou Q, Zhang B. Cold blood versus crystalloid cardioplegia for myocardial protection in adult cardiac surgery: a meta-analysis of randomized controlled studies. J. Cardiothorac. Vasc. Anesth. 2014 Jun;28(3):674-81.

184. Owen CM, Asopa S, Smart NA, King N. Microplegia in cardiac surgery: Systematic review and meta-analysis. J. Card. Surg. 2020 Oct;35(10):2737-46.

185. Schutz A, Zhang Q, Bertapelle K, Beecher N, Long W, Lee VV, et al. Del Nido cardioplegia in coronary surgery: a propensity-matched analysis. Interact. Cardiovasc. Thorac. Surg. 2020 May 1;30(5):699-705.

186 Mallidi HR, Sever J, Tamariz M, Singh S, Hanayama N, Christakis GT, et al. The short-term and long-term effects of warm or tepid cardioplegia. J. Thorac. Cardiovasc. Surg. 2003 Mar;125(3):711-20.

187. Allen BS, Winkelmann JW, Hanafy H, Hartz RS, Bolling KS, Ham J, Feinstein S. Retrograde cardioplegia does not adequately perfuse the right ventricle. J. Thorac. Cardiovasc. Surg. 1995 Jun;109(6):1116-24; discussion 24-6.

188. Candilio L, Malik A, Ariti C, Khan SA, Barnard M, Di Salvo C, et al. A retrospective analysis of myocardial preservation techniques during coronary artery bypass graft surgery: are we protecting the heart? J. Cardiothorac. Surg. 2014 Dec 31;9:184.

189. Ali M, Moeen M, Paras I, Hamid W, Khan S, Chaudhary MH. Cardio-Protective Effects of Multiport Antegrade Cold Blood Cardioplegia Versus Antegrade Cold Blood Cardioplegia in Patients With Left Ventricular Systolic Dysfunction Undergoing Conventional Coronary Artery Bypass Grafting. Curēus. 2020 Sep 8;12(9):e10308.

190. Radmehr H, Soleimani A, Tatari H, Salehi M. Does combined antegrade-retrograde cardioplegia have any superiority over antegrade cardioplegia? Heart Lung Circ. 2008 Dec;17(6):475-7.

191. Habertheuer A, Kocher A, Laufer G, Andreas M, Szeto WY, Petzelbauer P, et al. Cardioprotection: a review of current practice in global ischemia and future translational perspective. Biomed Res Int. 2014;2014:325725.

192. Guan Z, Guan X, Gu K, Lin X, Lin J, Zhou W, et al. Short-term outcomes of on- vs off-pump coronary artery bypass grafting in patients with left ventricular dysfunction: a systematic review and meta-analysis. J. Cardiothorac. Surg. 2020 May 11;15(1):84.

193. Shaefi S, Mittel A, Loberman D, Ramakrishna H. Off-Pump Versus On-Pump Coronary Artery Bypass Grafting-A Systematic Review and Analysis of Clinical Outcomes. J. Cardiothorac. Vasc. Anesth. 2019 Jan;33(1):232-44.

194. Zhu MZL, Huq MM, Billah BM, Tran L, Reid CM, Varatharajah K, Rosenfeldt FL. On-Pump Beating Heart Versus Conventional Coronary Artery Bypass Grafting Early After Myocardial Infarction: A Propensity-Score Matched Analysis From the ANZSCTS Database. Heart Lung Circ. 2019 Aug;28(8):1267-76.

195. Sheikhy A, Fallahzadeh A, Forouzannia K, Pashang M, Tajdini M, Momtahen S, et al. Off-pump versus on-pump coronary artery bypass graft surgery outcomes in patients with severe left ventricle dysfunction: inverse probability weighted study. BMC Cardiovasc. Disord. 2022 Nov 17;22(1):488.

196. Seese L, Sultan I, Wang Y, Navid F, Kilic A. Off-pump coronary artery bypass surgery lacks a longitudinal survival advantage in patients with left ventricular dysfunction. J. Card. Surg. 2020 Aug;35(8):1793-801.

197. Spetsotaki K, Zayat R, Donuru S, Autschbach R, Schnoering H, Hatam N. Evaluation of Left Ventricular Myocardial Work Performance in Patients Undergoing On-Pump and Off-Pump Coronary Artery Bypass Surgery. Ann Thorac Cardiovasc Surg. 2020 Oct 21;26(5):276-85.

198. Wang C, Chen J, Gu C, Li J. Analysis of survival after coronary endarterectomy combined with coronary artery bypass grafting compared with isolated coronary artery bypass grafting: a meta-analysis. Interact. Cardiovasc. Thorac. Surg. 2019 Sep 1;29(3):393-401.

199. Jiang R, Wang Y, Pang L, Sun X, Chu X, Wang F, Huang J. Feasibility of off-pump coronary artery grafting for patients with impaired left ventricular ejection fraction: A retrospective cohort study from a single institutional database. J. Card. Surg. 2021 Jun;36(6):1935-42.

200. Bonatti J, Wallner S, Crailsheim I, Grabenwoger M, Winkler B. Minimally invasive and robotic coronary artery bypass grafting-a 25-year review. J. Thorac. Dis. 2021 Mar;13(3):1922-44.

201. Gaudino M, Bakaeen F, Davierwala P, Di Franco A, Fremes SE, Patel N, et al. New Strategies for Surgical Myocardial Revascularization. Circulation. 2018 Nov 6;138(19):2160-8.

202. Shah PJ, Gordon I, Fuller J, Seevanayagam S, Rosalion A, Tatoulis J, et al. Factors affecting saphenous vein graft patency: clinical and angiographic study in 1402 symptomatic patients operated on between 1977 and 1999. J. Thorac. Cardiovasc. Surg. 2003 Dec;126(6):1972-7.

203. Caliskan E, de Souza DR, Boning A, Liakopoulos OJ, Choi YH, Pepper J, et al. Saphenous vein grafts in contemporary coronary artery bypass graft surgery. Nat. Rev. Cardiol. 2020 Mar;17(3):155-69.

204. Barner HB. The internal mammary artery as a free graft. J. Thorac. Cardiovasc. Surg. 1973 Aug;66(2):219-21.

205. Calafiore AM, Di Giammarco G, Luciani N, Maddestra N, Di Nardo E, Angelini R. Composite arterial conduits for a wider arterial myocardial revascularization. Ann. Thorac. Surg. 1994 Jul;58(1):185-90.

206. Bical O, Braunberger E, Fischer M, Robinault J, Foiret JC, Fromes Y, et al. Bilateral skeletonized mammary artery grafting: experience with 560 consecutive patients. Eur. J. Cardiothorac. Surg. 1996;10(11):971-5; discussion 6.

207. Dion R, Verhelst R, Rousseau M, Goenen M, Ponlot R, Kestens-Servaye Y, Chalant CH. Sequential mammary grafting. Clinical, functional, and angiographic assessment 6 months postoperatively in 231 consecutive patients. J. Thorac. Cardiovasc. Surg. 1989 Jul;98(1):80-8; discussion 8-9.

208. Gaudino M, Alessandrini F, Pragliola C, Luciani N, Trani C, Burzotta F, et al. Composite Y internal thoracic artery-saphenous vein grafts: short-term angiographic results and vasoreactive profile. J. Thorac. Cardiovasc. Surg. 2004 Apr;127(4):1139-44.

209. Buxton BF, Hayward PA, Newcomb AE, Moten S, Seevanayagam S, Gordon I. Choice of conduits for coronary artery bypass grafting: craft or science? Eur. J. Cardiothorac. Surg. 2009 Apr;35(4):658-70.

210. Buxton BF, Ruengsakulrach P, Fuller J, Rosalion A, Reid CM, Tatoulis J. The right internal thoracic artery graft--benefits of grafting the left coronary system and native vessels with a high grade stenosis. Eur. J. Cardiothorac. Surg. 2000 Sep;18(3):255-61.

211. Kim MS, Hwang HY, Kim JS, Oh SJ, Jang MJ, Kim KB. Saphenous vein versus right internal thoracic artery as a Y-composite graft: Five-year angiographic and clinical results of a randomized trial. J. Thorac. Cardiovasc. Surg. 2018 Oct;156(4):1424-33 e1.

212. Serruys PW, Morice MC, Kappetein AP, Colombo A, Holmes DR, Mack MJ, et al. Percutaneous coronary intervention versus coronary-artery bypass grafting for severe coronary artery disease. N. Engl. J. Med. 2009 Mar 5;360(10):961-72.

213. Pretto P, Martins GF, Biscaro A, Kruczan DD, Jessen B. Perioperative myocardial infarction in patients undergoing myocardial revascularization surgery. Rev. Bras. Cir. Cardiovasc. 2015 Jan-Mar;30(1):49-54.

214. Lomivorotov VV, Efremov SM, Kirov MY, Fominskiy EV, Karaskov AM. Low-Cardiac-Output Syndrome After Cardiac Surgery. J. Cardiothorac. Vasc. Anesth. 2017 Feb;31(1):291-308.

215. Sa MP, Nogueira JR, Ferraz PE, Figueiredo OJ, Cavalcante WC, Cavalcante TC, et al. Risk factors for low cardiac output syndrome after coronary artery bypass grafting surgery. Rev. Bras. Cir. Cardiovasc. 2012 Apr-Jun;27(2):217-23.

216. Nielsen DV, Hansen MK, Johnsen SP, Hansen M, Hindsholm K, Jakobsen C-J. Health outcomes with and without use of inotropic therapy in cardiac surgery: results of a propensity score-matched analysis. Anesthesiology. 2014;120(5):1098-108.

217. Yoon YH, Ahn JM, Kang DY, Park H, Cho SC, Lee PH, et al. Impact of SYNTAX Score on 10-Year Outcomes After Revascularization for Left Main Coronary Artery Disease. JACC Cardiovasc. Interv. 2020 Feb 10;13(3):361-71.

218. Eriksson HI, Jalonen JR, Heikkinen LO, Kivikko M, Laine M, Leino KA, et al. Levosimendan facilitates weaning from cardiopulmonary bypass in patients undergoing coronary artery bypass grafting with impaired left ventricular function. Ann. Thorac. Surg. 2009 Feb;87(2):448-54.

219. Tritapepe L, De Santis V, Vitale D, Guarracino F, Pellegrini F, Pietropaoli P, Singer M. Levosimendan pre-treatment improves outcomes in patients undergoing coronary artery bypass graft surgery. Br. J. Anaesth. 2009 Feb;102(2):198-204.

220 Levin R, Degrange M, Del Mazo C, Tanus E, Porcile R. Preoperative levosimendan decreases mortality and the development of low cardiac output in high-risk patients with severe left ventricular dysfunction undergoing coronary artery bypass grafting with cardiopulmonary bypass. Exp. Clin. Cardiol. 2012 Sep;17(3):125-30.

221. van Diepen S, Mehta RH, Leimberger JD, Goodman SG, Fremes S, Jankowich R, et al. Levosimendan in patients with reduced left ventricular function undergoing isolated coronary or valve surgery. J. Thorac. Cardiovasc. Surg. 2020 Jun;159(6):2302-9 e6.

222. JL M. Is epsilon aminocaproic acid as effective as aprotinin in reducing bleeding with cardiac surgery. Circulation. 1999;99:81-9.

223. Karthik S, Grayson AD, McCarron EE, Pullan DM, Desmond MJ. Reexploration for bleeding after coronary artery bypass surgery: risk factors, outcomes, and the effect of time delay. Ann. Thorac. Surg. 2004 Aug;78(2):527-34; discussion 34.

224. Mehta RH, Sheng S, O'Brien SM, Grover FL, Gammie JS, Ferguson TB, et al. Reoperation for bleeding in patients undergoing coronary artery bypass surgery: incidence, risk factors, time trends, and outcomes. Circ. Cardiovasc. Qual. Outcomes. 2009 Nov;2(6):583-90.

225. Ruel MA, Rubens FD. Non-pharmacological strategies for blood conservation in cardiac surgery. Can. J. Anaesth. 2001 Apr;48(4 Suppl):S13-23.

226. Horwich P, Buth KJ, Légaré JF. New onset postoperative atrial fibrillation is associated with a long-term risk for stroke and death following cardiac surgery. Journal of Cardiac Surgery: Including Mechanical and Biological Support for the Heart and Lungs. 2013;28(1):8-13.

227. Mariscalco G, Biancari F, Zanobini M, Cottini M, Piffaretti G, Saccocci M, et al. Bedside tool for predicting the risk of postoperative atrial fibrillation after cardiac surgery: the POAF score. J. Am. Coll. Cardiol. 2014 Mar 24;3(2):e000752.

228. Hogue CW, Jr, Palin CA, Arrowsmith JE. Cardiopulmonary bypass management and neurologic outcomes: an evidence-based appraisal of current practices. Anesth. Analg. 2006 Jul;103(1):21-37.

229. Echahidi N, Pibarot P, O'Hara G, Mathieu P. Mechanisms, prevention, and treatment of atrial fibrillation after cardiac surgery. J. Am. Coll. Cardiol. 2008 Feb 26;51(8):793-801.

230. Tsai YT, Lai CH, Loh SH, Lin CY, Lin YC, Lee CY, et al. Assessment of the Risk Factors and Outcomes for Postoperative Atrial Fibrillation Patients Undergoing Isolated Coronary Artery Bypass Grafting. Acta Cardiol Sin. 2015 Sep;31(5):436-43.

231. El-Chami MF, Kilgo P, Thourani V, Lattouf OM, Delurgio DB, Guyton RA, et al. New-onset atrial fibrillation predicts long-term mortality after coronary artery bypass graft. J. Am. Coll. Cardiol. 2010 Mar 30;55(13):1370-6.

232. Sadr-Ameli MA, Alizadeh A, Ghasemi V, Heidarali M. Ventricular tachyarrhythmia after coronary bypass surgery: incidence and outcome. Asian Cardiovasc. Thorac. Ann. 2013 Oct;21(5):551-7.

233. Lepelletier D, Perron S, Michaud J. Mediastinitis after cardiac surgery: incidence, microbiology and risk factors. Antibiotiques. 2005;7(1):18-22.

234. Lemaignen A, Birgand G, Ghodhbane W, Alkhoder S, Lolom I, Belorgey S, et al. Sternal wound infection after cardiac surgery: incidence and risk factors according to clinical presentation. Clin. Microbiol. Infect. 2015 Jul;21(7):674 e11-8.

235. Beaubien-Souligny W. Acute congestive renal failure in cardiac surgery [Thesis: Thèse de sciences]: Université de Montréal; 2021.

236. Dardashti A, Ederoth P, Algotsson L, Bronden B, Bjursten H. Incidence, dynamics, and prognostic value of acute kidney injury for death after cardiac surgery. J. Thorac. Cardiovasc. Surg. 2014 Feb;147(2):800-7.

237. Bahar I, Akgul A, Ozatik MA, Vural KM, Demirbag AE, Boran M, Tasdemir O. Acute renal failure following open heart surgery: risk factors and prognosis. Perfusion. 2005 Oct;20(6):317-22.

238. Nigwekar SU, Kandula P, Hix JK, Thakar CV. Off-pump coronary artery bypass surgery and acute kidney injury: a meta-analysis of randomized and observational studies. Am. J. Kidney Dis. 2009 Sep;54(3):413-23.

239. Landoni G, Bove T, Crivellari M, Poli D, Fochi O, Marchetti C, et al. Acute renal failure after isolated CABG surgery: six years of experience. Minerva Anestesiol. 2007 Nov;73(11):559-65.

240. Sirvinskas E, Andrejaitiene J, Raliene L, Nasvytis L, Karbonskiene A, Pilvinis V, Sakalauskas J. Cardiopulmonary bypass management and acute renal failure: risk factors and prognosis. Perfusion. 2008 Nov;23(6):323-7.

241. Rodrigues AJ, Evora PR, Bassetto S, Alves Junior L, Scorzoni Filho A, Araujo WF, Vicente WV. Risk factors for acute renal failure after heart surgery. Rev. Bras. Cir. Cardiovasc. 2009 Oct-Dec;24(4):441-6.

242. Karkouti K, Wijeysundera DN, Yau TM, Callum JL, Cheng DC, Crowther M, et al. Acute kidney injury after cardiac surgery: focus on modifiable risk factors. Circulation. 2009 Feb 3;119(4):495-502.

243. Macedo E, Malhotra R, Claure-Del Granado R, Fedullo P, Mehta RL. Defining urine output criterion for acute kidney injury in critically ill patients. Nephrol. Dial. Transplant. 2011 Feb;26(2):509-15.

244. Candela-Toha A, Elias-Martin E, Abraira V, Tenorio MT, Parise D, de Pablo A, et al. Predicting acute renal failure after cardiac surgery: external validation of two new clinical scores. Clin. J. Am. Soc. Nephrol. 2008 Sep;3(5):1260-5.

245. Birnie K, Verheyden V, Pagano D, Bhabra M, Tilling K, Sterne JA, Murphy GJ. Predictive models for kidney disease: improving global outcomes (KDIGO) defined acute kidney injury in UK cardiac surgery. Critical Care. 2014 2014/11/20;18(6):606.

246. Fischer UM, Weissenberger WK, Warters RD, Geissler HJ, Allen SJ, Mehlhorn U. Impact of cardiopulmonary bypass management on postcardiac surgery renal function. Perfusion. 2002 Nov;17(6):401-6.

247. Kumar AB, Suneja M, Bayman EO, Weide GD, Tarasi M. Association between postoperative acute kidney injury and duration of cardiopulmonary bypass: a meta-analysis. J. Cardiothorac. Vasc. Anesth. 2012;26(1):64-9.

248. Chawla LS, Zhao Y, Lough FC, Schroeder E, Seneff MG, Brennan JM. Off-pump versus on-pump coronary artery bypass grafting outcomes stratified by preoperative renal function. J. Am. Soc. Nephrol. 2012 Aug;23(8):1389-97.

249. Lamy A, Devereaux P, Prabhakaran D, Taggart DP, Hu S, Paolasso E, et al. Off-pump or on-pump coronary-artery bypass grafting at 30 days. N. Engl. J. Med. 2012;366(16):1489-97.

250. Bax JJ, Maddahi J, Poldermans D, Elhendy A, Schinkel A, Boersma E, et al. Preoperative comparison of different noninvasive strategies for predicting improvement in left ventricular function after coronary artery bypass grafting. Am. J. Cardiol. 2003 Jul 1;92(1):1-4.

251. Carluccio E, Biagioli P, Alunni G, Murrone A, Giombolini C, Ragni T, et al. Patients with hibernating myocardium show altered left ventricular volumes and shape, which revert after revascularization: evidence that dyssynergy might directly induce cardiac remodeling. J. Am. Coll. Cardiol. 2006;47(5):969-77.

252. Soraas CL, Larstorp AC, Mangschau A, Tonnessen T, Kjeldsen SE, Bjornerheim R. Echocardiographic demonstration of improved myocardial function early after coronary artery bypass graft surgery. Interact. Cardiovasc. Thorac. Surg. 2011 Jun;12(6):946-51.

253. Knapp M, Musial WJ, Lisowska A, Hirnle T. The value of dobutamine stress echocardiography in predicting clinical improvement following coronary artery bypass grafting in patients with left ventricular systolic dysfunction. Cardiol J. 2007;14(2):174-9.

254. Garzillo CL, Hueb W, Gersh BJ, Lima EG, Rezende PC, Hueb AC, et al. Long-term analysis of left ventricular ejection fraction in patients with stable multivessel coronary disease undergoing medicine, angioplasty or surgery: 10-year follow-up of the MASS II trial. Eur. Heart J. 2013 Nov;34(43):3370-7.

255. Bax JJ, Visser FC, Poldermans D, Elhendy A, Cornel JH, Boersma E, et al. Time course of functional recovery of stunned and hibernating segments after surgical revascularization. Circulation. 2001 Sep 18;104(12 Suppl 1):I314-8.

256. Carr JA, Haithcock BE, Paone G, Bernabei AF, Silverman NA. Long-term outcome after coronary artery bypass grafting in patients with severe left ventricular dysfunction. Ann. Thorac. Surg. 2002 Nov;74(5):1531-6.

257. Lee S, Chang BC, Yoo KJ, Hong YS, Kang MS. Clinical results of coronary revascularization in left ventricular dysfunction. Circ. J. 2007 Dec;71(12):1862-6.

258. Basiladze L, Prangishvili A, Chapidze G, Pirvelashvili E, Bakhutashvili Z. Coronary artery bypass grafting in patients with low ejection fraction. Georgian Med. News. 2009 Nov;176(176):17-21.

259. Hamad MS, Peels K, Van Straten A, Van Zundert A, Schonberger J. Coronary artery bypass surgery in patients with impaired left ventricular function. Predictors of hospital outcome. Acta Anaesthesiol. Belg. 2006;58(1):37.

260 Uyar IS, Sahin V, Akpinar MB, Abacilar F, Yurtman V, Okur FF, et al. editors. Decision making and results of coronary artery bypass grafting for patients with poor left ventricular function. The Heart Surgery Forum; 2013.

261. Herlitz J, Karlson BW, Sjoland H, Brandrup-Wognsen G, Haglid M, Karlsson T, Caidahl K. Long term prognosis after CABG in relation to preoperative left ventricular ejection fraction. Int. J. Cardiol. 2000 Jan 15;72(2):163-71; discussion 73-4.

Appendices

APPENDIX 1: Data collection form

Data collection media

First and last name:
....
......
File number:
....
......
Date of birth:
....
......
Pre-operation data :
Age: 1. <40 2. 40-50 3. 50-60 4. >60
Sex: 1.male 2. Female
Coronary heredity: 1. Yes 2. No
IMC: 1. <30 2. >30
HTA: 1. yes 2. No
Diabetes: 1. yes 2. no No
Type of diabetes: 1. T2DM 2. NIDDM 3. Insulin dependent 4. First discovered
Dyslipidemia: 1. Yes 2. No
Sedentary lifestyle: 1. Yes 2. No
Smoking: 1. yes 2. no No
Redux: 1. yes 2. No
Coronary history: 1. Medical treatment 2. Angioplasty 3. Bypass surgery
Peripheral arteriopathy: 1. yes 2. no No
Symptomatology of ACOMI: 1. intermittent claudication 2. Rest pain
3. Critical ischemia
TTT for ACOMI: 1. Medical 2. Surgical
Carotid stenosis: 1. Yes 2. No
Degrees of carotid stenosis: 1. <70% 2. > 70% 3. >80%
Treatment of carotid stenosis: 1. Medical 2. Surgical
Stroke: 1. yes 2. No
TIA: 1. yes 2. No
Type of stroke: 1. Ischemic 2. Hemorrhagic
Neurological sequelae: 1. yes 2. no No
Renal insufficiency: 1. Yes 2. No
Creatinine clearance value: ....
Creatinine clearance: 1. >=90 2. 60-89 3. 30-59 4.15-29 5. <15

COPD: 1. Yes 2. No
Emergency: 1. Yes 2. No
Degrees of urgency: 1. TV 2. Counterpulsation balloon 3. Recovered cardiac arrest 4. pre-operative mechanical ventilation 5. Vasopressor agents 6. acute renal failure
Hemodynamically unstable: 1. yes 2. no No
NYHA : 1. I 2. II 3. III 4. IV
Orthopnea: 1. yes 2. no No
IMO: 1. Yes 2. No
Syncope: 1. yes 2. no No
Lipothymia: 1. yes 2. no No
IVG flare-up: 1. yes 2. No
Stress angina: 1. Yes 2. No
SCA: 1. ST + 2. ST -
ACS: 1. With troponin elevation 2. Without troponin elevation
Other reason for consultation: 1. Yes 2. No
Description:
....
Stress test: 1. Yes 2. No
Myocardial scintigraphy: 1. yes 2. no No
Recent MI: 1.Yes 2. No
Clopidogrel: 1. yes 2. no No
Aspégic : 1. Yes 2. No
Anti-GP IIB IIIA: 1. yes 2. no No
UFH: 1. yes 2. No
LMWH: 1. yes 2. No
AVK: 1. yes 2. No
Cordarone: 1. yes 2. No
Digoxin: 1. yes 2.no
B blocking: 1. Yes 2. No
Diuretic: 1. yes 2. no No
IEC: 1. Yes 2. No
SCBA II: 1. yes 2. No
Calcium inhibitor: 1. Yes 2. No
Nitro derivative: 1. Yes 2. No
Statin: 1. Yes 2. No
Chest X-ray:
....
....
ECG data :
Cardiac rhythm: 1. Sinus 2. ACFA 3. BAV 4. BBG
Repolarization disorders: 1. ST shift 2. ST undershift 3. Necrosis Q wave
4. Negative T wave 5. Normal

Biology :

Hb: .... Hte : .... GB : .... PQ : ....

Troponin: 1. Positive 2. Negative

Preoperative ETT data:

LVEF: ....

PAH: 1. yes 2. No

PAPS value: ....

Disturbance of segmental kinetics: 1. yes 2. no No

Description:

....

Associated valve disease: 1. Yes 2. No

Type of valve disease: ....

Coronary angiography :

Location of TCG stenosis: 1. Proximal 2. Intermediate 3. Distal 4. Tubular

Type of stenosis: 1. Tight (50-69%) 2. Very tight (70-89%) 3. Critical (>=90%)

Status: 1. Monotruncular 2. Bi-truncular 3. Tritruncular

Stenotic arteries: 1. IVA 2. Bx 3. CX 4. CD 5. Dg 6. Mg 7. IVP 8. RVG

Types of stenosis for each artery: 1. Intermediate 2. Tight 3. Very tight

Stented artery: 1. Yes 2. No ....

Bridged artery: 1. Yes 2. No ....

Occluded artery: 1. IVA 2. Bx 3. CX 4. CD 5. Dg 6. Mg 7. IVP 8. RVG

Time to revascularization: ....

Time to revascularization: 1. 2-4d 2. 5-8d 3. 9-15d 4. 16-30d 5. >30j

Levosimendan: 1. Yes 2. No

ASA: 1. I 2. II 3. III 4. IV 5. V

Euroscore II:

....

Euroscore II: 1. <5% 2. 5-10% 3. >10%

STS scores: Risk of mortality: ....

Morbidity or mortality: ....

Intraoperative data :

PAC : 1. CEC 2. Beating heart 3. CB conversion to CEC

Act: 1. Single PAC 2. Double PAC 3. Triple PAC 4. Quad PAC 5. Quintuple PAC

Grafters: 1. AMIG 2. Sequential mammary 3. Double mammary 4. Mammary + VSI 5. 2 mammaries + VSI

Grafting diagram:

....

Complete revascularization: 1. Yes 2. No

CEC data :

CEC duration:

....

....

Aortic clamping time:

....

Support period:

....

....

Cardioplegia route: 1. Anterograde 2. Retrograde 3. Mixed

Type of cardioplegia: 1. Blood 2. Crystalloid 3. Blood + crystalloid 4. Other

Quantity of cardioplegia: 1. 1 dose 1. 1 dose +1/2 2. 2 doses 3. 3 doses 4. > 3 doses

Vasopressor agents: 1. NAD 2. Dobu 3. NAD + Dobu 4. Adré 5. Nothing

Ventricular fibrillation: 1. yes 2. no No

Internal electric shock: 1. Yes 2. No

ACFA : 1. yes 2. No

Temporary pacing: 1. Bradycardia 2. BAV

Dependence on external stimulation: 1. Yes 2. No

CEC exit: 1. Easy 2. High doses of catecholamines 3. Assistance 4. Resuming bypass surgery

5. Counter-pulse ball

Transfusion: 1. Yes 2. No

Intraoperative death: 1. Yes 2. No

Postoperative data :

Duration of mechanical ventilation: ....h

Extubation <6h: 1. Yes 2. No

Length of stay in intensive care unit: 1. 1 d 2. 2 d 3. 3 d 4. > 3 j

....

Length of stay in hospital: 1. 3 d 2. 4 d 3. 5 d 4. 6 d 5. 7 d 6. >7 j

....

Biology :

Early postoperative TTE:

LVEF: ....

LVEF: 1. Improved 2. Same as 3. Altered

PAPS: ....

PAPS : 1. <=30 2. >30

Disturbances in kinetics: 1. yes 2. no No

Postoperative complications:

Hemorrhage :

Bleeding (> 150 ml /4 first hours): 1. yes 2. no No

Quantity: ....

Resume: 1. yes 2. No
Transfusion: 1. Yes 2. No
CGR: ....
PFC: ....
PQ: ....
Fibrinogen: 1. Yes 2. No
Factor VII: 1. Yes 2. No
Exacyl: 1. yes 2. No
Hemorrhagic shock: 1. Yes 2. No
Digestive bleeding: 1. yes 2. no No
Cardiovascular :
Low cardiac output: 1. Yes 2. No
Counter-pulse ball: 1. Yes 2. No
IDM : 1. yes 2. No
Clopidogrel: 1. yes 2. no No
Cardiogenic OAP: 1. Yes 2. No
Ischemic stroke: 1. yes 2. no No
Hemorrhagic stroke: 1. yes 2. no No
ECMO: 1. yes 2. No
Tonicardiacs: 1. NAD 2. Dobu 3. NAD+ Dobu 4. Adré 5. Nothing
Supraventricular arrhythmia: 1. Yes 2. No
Auriculoventricular boc: 1. yes 2. no No
Pericardial effusion: 1. Yes 2. No
Tamponnade: 1. yes 2. No
Respiratory complications :
ARDS: 1. Yes 2. No
Use of NIV: 1. Yes 2. No
Re intubation: 1. Yes 2. Yes
Prolonged mechanical ventilation: 1. Yes 2. No
Mechanical ventilation: ....h
Pulmonary embolism: 1. yes 2. no No
Curative anticoagulation: 1. Yes 2. No
PNO: 1. yes 2. No
Infectious complications :
Mediastinitis: 1. Yes 2. No
Resume: 1. yes 2. No
Return time: ....
Bronchopulmonary infection: 1. yes 2. no No
Urinary tract infection: 1. yes 2. no No
Sepsis: 1. yes 2. no No
Septic shock: 1. Yes 2. No
TBA: 1. Yes 2. No

ATB:
....
....

Renal complications :

Postoperative renal failure: 1. yes 2. no No
Postoperative creatinine clearance:
....
...

Hemodialysis: 1. yes 2. no No
Hepatic cytolysis: 1. yes 2. no No
Transfusion accident: 1. Yes 2. No
Multivisceral failure: 1. Yes 2. No
Death: 1. yes 2. no No

Cardiology follow-up: more than 2 years :

ETT :

1er follow-up: ....months

LVEF:
....
LVEF: 1. Improved 2. Same as 3. Altered
PAPS: 1. <=30 2. >30 value:...
Kinetics disorder: 1. yes 2. no No

2ème follow-up: ....months

LVEF:
....
LVEF: 1. Improved 2. Same as 3. Altered
PAPS: 1. <=30 2. >30 value:...
Kinetics disorder: 1. yes 2. no No

3ème follow-up: ....months

LVEF:
....
LVEF: 1. Improved 2. Same as 3. Altered
PAPS: 1. <=30 2. >30 value:...
Kinetics disorder: 1. yes 2. no No

Mortality: 1. Yes 2. No
Time to death: ....

Clinical :

Asymptomatic: 1. Yes 2. No
Symptomatology:
....
....
SCA: 1. yes 2. No

Residual angina: 1. Yes 2. No
Dyspnea: 1. Yes 2. No
NYHA : 1. I 2. II 3. III 4. IV 5. V
Stroke: 1. yes 2. No
Acute congestive heart failure: 1. Yes 2. No
ECG: repolarization disorders: 1. Yes 2. No
ACFA: 1. yes 2. No
Coronary angiography :
....
....
....
Angioplasty: 1. Yes 2. No
....
....
....

APPENDIX 2: NYHA classification

Class	Clinical expression
Class I	patients with no limitation of ordinary activities
Class II	mild activity limitation
Class III	marked limitation of activity, they are more at ease than at rest
Class IV	symptoms occur even at rest

APPENDIX 3: Coronary flow and TIMI score

- Le flux TIMI 0 : c'est l'occlusion. Aucun produit de contraste ne passe à travers la sténose
- Le flux TIMI 1 : le contraste passe à travers la sténose mais n'opacifie pas complètement le lit d'aval
- Le flux TIMI 2 : le contraste passe la sténose mais il y a un retard de flux en aval de la sténose
- Le flux TIMI 3 : flux normal, identique en aval qu'en amont de la sténose

APPENDIX 4: ASA Physical Status Classification System

1: Normal patient
2: Patient with moderate systemic abnormality
3: Patient with severe systemic abnormality
4: Patient with severe systemic abnormality representing a constant life threat
5: Moribund patient unlikely to survive without intervention
6 : Patient declared brain dead whose organs are removed for transplantation

APPENDIX 5:EuroSCORE II calculator

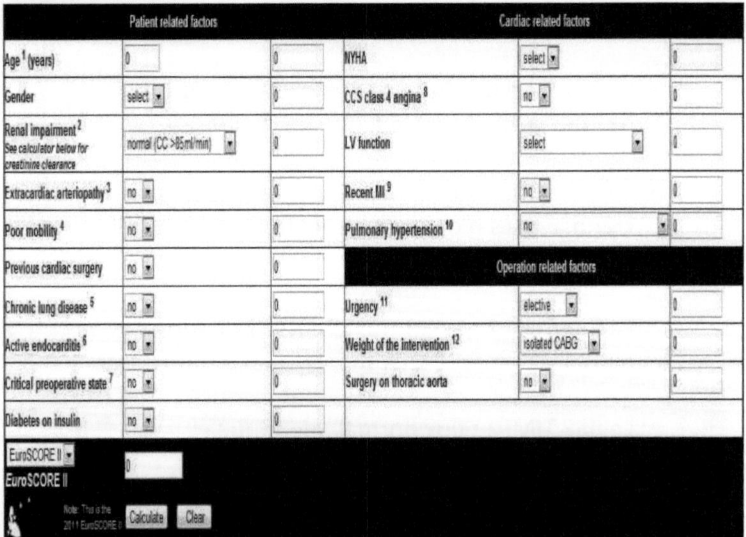

Patient related factors			Cardiac related factors		
Age [1] (years)	0	0	NYHA	select	0
Gender	select	0	CCS class 4 angina [8]	no	0
Renal impairment [2] See calculator below for creatinine clearance	normal (CC >85ml/min)	0	LV function	select	0
Extracardiac arteriopathy [3]	no	0	Recent MI [9]	no	0
Poor mobility [4]	no	0	Pulmonary hypertension [10]	no	0
Previous cardiac surgery	no	0	Operation related factors		
Chronic lung disease [5]	no	0	Urgency [11]	elective	0
Active endocarditis [6]	no	0	Weight of the intervention [12]	isolated CABG	0
Critical preoperative state [7]	no	0	Surgery on thoracic aorta	no	0
Diabetes on insulin	no	0			
EuroSCORE II EuroSCORE II Note: This is the 2011 EuroSCORE II	0 Calculate Clear				

APPENDIX 6:STS Risk Score calculator

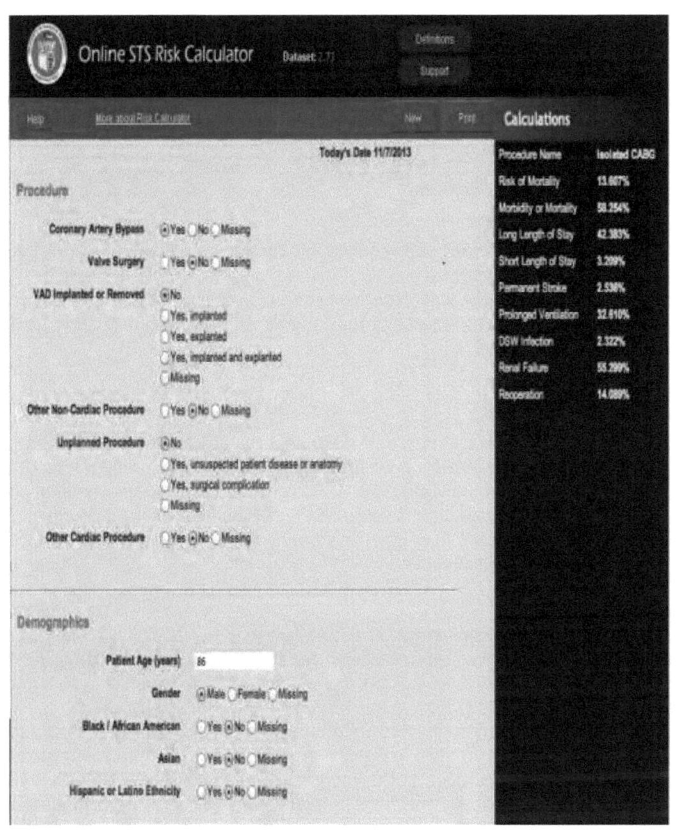

Online STS Risk Calculator
Dataset: 2.73
Definitions
Support
Help
More about Risk Calculator
New
Print
Calculations
Today's Date 11/7/2013
Procedure
Coronary Artery Bypass Yes No Missing
Valve Surgery Yes No Missing
VAD Implanted or Removed No
Yes, implanted
Yes, explanted
Yes, implanted and explanted
Missing
Other Non-Cardiac Procedure Yes No Missing
Unplanned Procedure No
Yes, unsuspected patient disease or anatomy
Yes, surgical complication
Missing
Other Cardiac Procedure Yes No Missing
Demographics
Patient Age (years) 86
Gender Male Female Missing
Black / African American Yes No Missing
Asian Yes No Missing
Hispanic or Latino Ethnicity Yes No Missing
Procedure Name Isolated CABG
Risk of Mortality 13.607%
Morbidity or Mortality 58.254%
Long Length of Stay 42.383%
Short Length of Stay 3.209%
Permanent Stroke 2.536%
Prolonged Ventilation 32.610%
DSW Infection 2.322%
Renal Failure 55.299%
Reoperation 14.089%

SURGICAL REVASCULARIZATION IN PATIENTS WITH LEFT VENTRICULAR DYSFUNCTION: AN ANALYSIS OF OPERATIVE AND MID-TERM MORTALITY OUTCOMES

Abstract

Background:
For complex coronary disease and reduced left ventricular ejection fraction (LVEF), guidelines recommend coronary artery bypass grafting (CABG). However, this procedure has a high risk of postoperative mortality and morbidity. This study aimed to investigate morbidity and mortality for patients with a reduced ejection fraction LVEF ≤40%.

Methods:
We conducted a retrospective descriptive study at the Military Hospital of Tunis from 2012 to 2021, focusing on on-pump CABG patients with a preoperative LVEF ≤40%. Non-inclusion criteria were prior CABG or valvular heart replacements and myocardial infarction complications surgeries. Exclusion criteria included off-pump CABG, incomplete data, or follow-up. The study endpoints were the operative (≤30 days) and follow-up morbidity.

Results:
Seventy-three patients were included. The average age was 60 ± 7 years. Early postoperative major adverse cardiovascular events (MACCE) included deaths (22%), low cardiac output syndrome (LCOS) (38%), myocardial infarction (16%), and cerebrovascular accidents (1%).
Predictors of operative mortality were chronic lower limb arterial disease, chronic kidney disease (CKD), left main coronary artery disease, incomplete myocardial revascularization, postoperative LCOS, myocardial infarctions, postoperative acute kidney injury or infections, mechanical ventilation duration >10 hours, and postoperative LVEF ≤ 33%.
The median follow-up was eight years. Predictors of mortality during the follow-up were preoperative CKD, preoperative acute heart failure, Emergent CABG, preoperative antero-septal LV wall motion abnormalities, preoperative glycated hemoglobin ≥9%, mediastinitis, and a decrease in LVEF of more than five percent. An improvement in LVEF ≥5% was tethered to a less late mortality rate. Overall survival was 68.5% at two years and 57.9% at five years. In multivariate analysis, independent predictors of overall mortality were anterior or antero-septal LV wall motion abnormalities (OR=4.21), Emergent surgery (OR=1.1), and postoperative LCOS (OR=9.79).

Conclusion:
The observed morbidity and mortality reflect a significant operative risk of CABG in cases of reduced LVEF. Preoperative identification of mortality predictors by the medical-surgical team allows for risk assessment, anticipation of complications, and optimization of postoperative outcomes.

Keywords: Heart Failure, Coronary Artery Disease, Cardiac Surgery, Ventricular Dysfunction

SURGICAL REVASCULARIZATION OF CORONARY PATIENTS WITH LEFT VENTRICULAR DYSFUNCTION: STUDY OF IMMEDIATE AND MEDIUM-TERM MORTALITY

Summary

Introduction:

For complex coronary lesions, coronary artery bypass grafting (CABG) is the operation of choice despite its high postoperative morbi-mortality. The aim of this study was to investigate mortality in patients with preoperative LVEF ≤40%.

Methods :

This is a descriptive retrospective study conducted at the Tunis Military Hospital between 2012 and 2021 including patients undergoing CABG with LVEF≤40%. Concomitant prior cardiac or valvular surgeries as well as those treating a mechanical complication of myocardial infarction (MI) were not included. Incomplete records, lost to follow-up and beating heart surgery were excluded. Outcome measures were early mortality (<30 days) and late mortality post-PAC.

Results :

Seventy-three patients were included. The mean age was 60±7 years. Postoperatively, early major cardiovascular events(MACCE) were death(22%), low cardiac output syndrome(SBDC)(38%), MI (16%) and stroke (1%).

Predictors of early mortality were: chronic arterial disease of the lower limbs, chronic renal failure (CKD), common trunk stenosis, incomplete revascularization, intubation (VM) >10 hours, postoperative LVEF ≤ 33%, or a postoperative complication (SBDC, MI, acute renal failure or infection).

Median follow-up was eight years. Predictors of late mortality were: CKD, preoperative acute heart failure, surgery in extreme emergency, extensive preoperative anteroseptal hypokinesis, mediastinitis, preoperative glycated hemoglobin ≥9% or LVEF decline ≥5%. Conversely, improvement in LVEF ≥ 5% was associated with lower late mortality.

Overall survival was 69% at two years and 58% at five years. In multivariate analysis, the independent predictors of overall mortality were: anterior or anteroseptal kinetic disorders (OR=4.2), extreme emergency surgery (OR=1.1), and postoperative SBDC (OR=9.8).

Conclusion:

The morbi-mortality observed reflects a non-negligible operative risk of CABG in cases of reduced LVEF. Pre-operative detection of factors predictive of this morbi-mortality would enable better selection of patients in order to anticipate complications and optimize post-operative care.

Keywords: Heart failure , Coronary heart disease , Cardiac surgery , Ventricular dysfunction

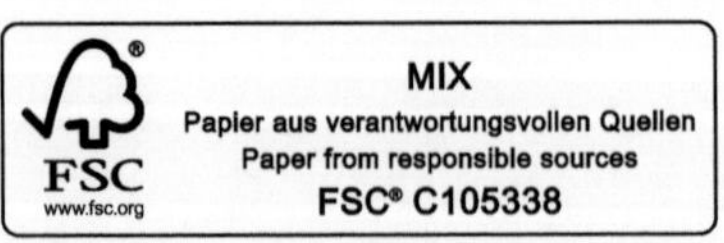

Printed by Books on Demand GmbH, Norderstedt / Germany